—— Essentials of ——

HEALTH JUSTICE

A PRIMER

ELIZABETH TOBIN-TYLER, JD, MA

Assistant Professor, Alpert Medical School
Brown University
Providence, Rhode Island

JOEL B. TEITELBAUM, JD, LLM

Department of Health Policy
Milken Institute School of Public Health
The George Washington University
Washington, DC

JONES & BARTLETT
LEARNING

World Headquarters
Jones & Bartlett Learning
5 Wall Street
Burlington, MA 01803
978-443-5000
info@jblearning.com
www.jblearning.com

Jones & Bartlett Learning books and products are available through most bookstores and online booksellers. To contact Jones & Bartlett Learning directly, call 800-832-0034, fax 978-443-8000, or visit our website, www.jblearning.com.

Substantial discounts on bulk quantities of Jones & Bartlett Learning publications are available to corporations, professional associations, and other qualified organizations. For details and specific discount information, contact the special sales department at Jones & Bartlett Learning via the above contact information or send an email to specialsales@jblearning.com.

Production Credits

VP, Product Management: David D. Cella
Director of Product Management: Michael Brown
Product Specialist: Danielle Bessette
Associate Production Editor: Alex Schab
Senior Marketing Manager: Sophie Fleck Teague
Production Services Manager: Colleen Lamy
Manufacturing and Inventory Control Supervisor: Amy Bacus
Composition: codeMantra U.S. LLC

Cover Design: Kristin E. Parker
Text Design: Kristin E. Parker
Director of Rights & Media: Joanna Gallant
Rights & Media Specialist: Merideth Tumasz
Media Development Editor: Shannon Sheehan
Cover Image (Title Page): © digitalskillet/Getty Images
Printing and Binding: Edwards Brothers Malloy
Cover Printing: Edwards Brothers Malloy

Library of Congress Cataloging-in-Publication Data
Names: Tyler, Elizabeth Tobin, author. | Teitelbaum, Joel Bern, author.
Title: Essentials of health justice: a primer / Elizabeth Tobin-Tyler and Joel B. Teitelbaum.
Description: Burlington, Massachusetts: Jones & Bartlett Learning, [2019] | Includes bibliographical references.
Identifiers: LCCN 2018003086 | ISBN 9781284152074 (paperback)
Subjects: | MESH: Healthcare Disparities | Social Determinants of Health | Vulnerable Populations | Social Justice | United States
Classification: LCC RA418 | NLM W 76 AA1 | DDC 362.1—dc23
LC record available at https://lccn.loc.gov/2018003086

6048

Printed in the United States of America
22 21 20 19 18   10 9 8 7 6 5 4 3 2 1

Contents

PART III Striving for Health Justice   91

Chapter 5 Safety Net Programs and Legal Protections That Support Health. 93

Chapter 6 Systems Change to Promote Health Equity 117

Chapter 7 Advocating for Health Justice: What You Can Do 147

Acknowledgments

We are grateful to several people who generously contributed their guidance and assistance to us during the writing of this text. At the top of the list are Dr. Richard Riegelman (founding dean of the now-called Milken Institute School of Public Health at the George Washington University and professor of epidemiology and biostatistics, medicine, and health policy) and Mike Brown (Director of Product Management for Jones & Bartlett Learning), who are spearheading an effort to create a series of books aimed at educating students across disciplines in the many facets of population health. We appreciate their vision in making health justice an integral part of that effort.

We also extend our deep thanks to the production staff at Jones & Bartlett Learning for their technical expertise and patience, and to Joanna Theiss, JD, LLM, for her stellar research assistance (and for safeguarding the local playgrounds!). We could not have brought this book to fruition without them.

Liz sends special thanks to John, Graham, Tobin, and Clare for their perpetual sustenance and encouragement and to her students and clinical and community partners who work so hard to achieve health justice. Joel sends special thanks to Laura, Jared, and Layna for their unique brand of alchemy, and to all the legal-aid lawyers, clinicians, and community workers who leverage the power of law to help lift up those in society whose life circumstances have other ideas.

About the Authors

Elizabeth Tobin-Tyler, JD, MA, is assistant professor of family medicine at the Alpert Medical School and assistant professor of health services, policy, and practice at the Brown University School of Public Health. She is co-director of the Health Systems Science I and II courses at the Alpert Medical School. She teaches, writes, and consults in the areas of health policy, health equity, public health law, and medical and public health ethics. Her research focuses on the role of law and policy in the social determinants of health, community-based, and health system interventions that address health disparities, and interprofessional medical-legal education.

Professor Tobin-Tyler is a national expert in the development of medical-legal partnerships, which integrate medicine, public health, and legal services to identify, address, and prevent health-harming social and legal needs of patients, clinics, and populations. She is senior editor and a contributor to the first textbook on the topic, *Poverty, Health and Law: Readings and Cases for Medical-Legal Partnership* (Carolina Academic Press, 2011). In 2013, she was awarded the Distinguished Advocate award by the National Center for Medical-Legal Partnership for her work in promoting the medical-legal partnership model and for developing interprofessional medical-legal education. In 2014, Professor Tobin-Tyler was selected as a Robert Wood Johnson Foundation Future of Public Health Law Education Faculty Fellow. She has served on a number of boards and advisory councils including the National Center for Medical-Legal Partnership board, the National Advisory Council for the Accelerating Interprofessional Community-Based Education and Practice Initiative, and the National Advisory Council for the Learning Collaborative on Health Equity and Young Children.

Joel B. Teitelbaum, JD, LLM, is an associate professor of health policy, director of the Hirsh Health Law and Policy Program, and co-director of the National Center for Medical-Legal Partnership, all at the George Washington University (GW) Milken Institute School of Public Health in Washington, DC. He also carries a faculty appointment with the GW Law School, and for 11 years he served as vice chair for academic affairs in the Department of Health Policy and Management.

Professor Teitelbaum has taught graduate courses on health care law, health care civil rights, public health law, minority health policy, and long-term care law and policy, and an undergraduate survey course on health law. He was the first member of the School of Public Health faculty to receive the university-wide Bender Teaching Award; he has received the school's Excellence in Teaching Award, and he is a member of the GW Academy of Distinguished Teachers. He has authored or co-authored dozens of articles, text chapters, policy papers, and reports on civil rights issues in health care, insurance law and policy, medical-legal partnership, health reform and its implementation, and behavioral health care quality, and he is co-author of *Essentials of Health Policy and Law, Third Edition* (2017), published by Jones & Bartlett Learning.

Among other organizations, Professor Teitelbaum is a member of Delta Omega, the national honor society recognizing excellence in the field of public health; the ASPH/Pfizer Public Health Academy of Distinguished Teachers; and the Society for American Law Teachers. In 2016, during President Obama's second term, Professor Teitelbaum was named to the U.S. Department of Health and Human Services Secretary's Advisory Committee on National Health Promotion and Disease Prevention Objectives for 2030 (i.e., Healthy People 2030). He also serves as special advisor to the American Bar Association's Commission on Veterans' Legal Services and as a member of the Board of Advisors of PREPARE, a national advanced care planning organization.

Introduction

Most population health experts would tell you that the global community lives in perilous times. Each of the following threatens the well-being of civilization, either in the here and now or in the not-too-distant future: climate change, food underproduction, overpopulation, epidemic disease (including multidrug-resistant "superbugs"), and emerging technologies such as biotechnology, nanotechnology, and artificial intelligence, all of which are becoming increasingly powerful and increasingly accessible to rogue governments and individuals alike. None of these threats can be addressed by any single nation or even by any particular region of the world. In our increasingly globalized existence—in which financial markets, labor, and other forms of migration, technology, and travel are becoming increasingly intertwined around the globe—most nations would need to embark on a truly concerted effort to prevent or reduce the major risks posed by these population health hazards. Even the United States, a world power by virtue of its military and economic clout, could do very little on its own to wipe out even one of the threats noted above, or to shield itself completely from their effects.

There is one invidious population health affliction, however, from which the U.S. already suffers and which actually is within the nation's power to control and remedy: health inequity. (This is not to say that health inequity is not a significant population health problem in other countries—it is, and its reduction is a priority in many countries. Our point is that here in the U.S., health inequity is neither a problem on the horizon nor one that requires a multinational response—it is an existing problem of our own making and one which we could solve independently.) One can find many definitions of *health equity*, but for purposes of this text we offer the following one: "Health equity means that everyone has a fair and just opportunity to be healthy. This requires removing obstacles to health, such as poverty, discrimination, and their consequences, including powerlessness and lack of access to good jobs with fair pay, quality education and housing, safe environments, and health care."[1] We selected this definition because we believe it succinctly encompasses many of the things discussed throughout this text: acknowledging historical and contemporary discrimination, valuing all people equally, focusing societal efforts on addressing avoidable injustices, and eliminating health and health care disparities. To get a sense of just how long health inequities have plagued our society, consider what you know about the colonists' treatment of Native Americans and about the enslavement of the millions of African people who were kidnapped and shipped to the Americas; do you think those Native Americans and Africans were given "a fair and just opportunity to be healthy"?

Before contextualizing and describing more fully the contents of this text, it is instructive to define and distinguish three other terms: *health equality, health disparity,* and *health care disparity*. Health equality is the absence of avoidable or remediable differences in health and health care among groups of people. To put it differently, health *in*equalities are "differences in health status or in the distribution of health determinants between different population groups."[2] The important difference between health equity and health equality is summed up nicely this way: "The nation's focus should be on achieving equity, not equality. One is a moral and fiscal imperative; the other is impossible. Because life choices, chance, and providence bring fortune and misfortune, no society can promise equal outcomes, and inequalities are inevitable. Furthermore, unequal health outcomes are not inherently unjust: They can arise from biology, personal choices, or chance."[3]

Separate from, but related to, health inequities and inequalities are health and health care disparities. A health disparity is a difference in health status that is closely linked with social, economic, and/or environmental disadvantage. In other words, these are health differences that exist between groups of people who have systematically experienced greater obstacles to health based on their race, ethnicity, religion, socioeconomic status, gender, age, mental or physical disability, sexual orientation or gender identity, or geographic location when compared with majority populations.[4] Health care disparities, on the other hand, refer to "differences in the *quality* of health care provided that are not due to access-related factors or clinical needs, preferences, and appropriateness of interventions. These differences would include the role of bias, discrimination, and stereotyping at the individual (provider and patient), institutional, and health system levels."[5]

Finally, recognize that we use yet another term—*health justice*—for the title of this text. "Justice" is defined by a typical dictionary as "just behavior or treatment," and as having "a concern for justice, peace, and genuine respect for people." Typical synonyms include fairness, evenhandedness, impartiality, and morality. While we could easily have used *health equity* in the book title, we settled on *health justice* because it tends to be relatively more recognized and understood by a greater number of people. For example, complete the following sentence in your mind: "I appealed to his sense of _____." Chances are you completed that sentence with either "justice" or "fairness", but not with "equity." Furthermore, "justice" is often linked in people's minds to the legal system, and we discuss at many points in this text the role of law in both creating and remediating health injustices. Thus, because we wanted this text to be as relatable as possible across a range of fields and disciplines, and because of the link between justice and legal recourse, we selected *health justice* for the title. If you're looking for a definition of health justice to hold onto as you read further, think of it simply as laws, policies, systems, and behaviors that are evenhanded with regard to and display genuine respect for *everyone's* health and well-being.

This Introduction contextualizes the concept of health justice by touching briefly on four overarching topics, all of which are more fully discussed at later points:

1. There is no across-the-board right to health, health care services, or health insurance in the U.S.
2. Social factors play a critical role in individual and population health.
3. Wealth equals health—and the U.S. currently faces historically high levels of economic inequality.
4. Society is too willing to medicalize social needs and criminalize social deficiencies.

After providing a summary of each of these topics, this Introduction concludes by describing the rationale for and structure of *Essentials of Health Justice: A Primer.*

▶ No Generalized Right to Health, Health Care, or Health Insurance

An obvious starting point for an introductory section on health justice is the fact that in the U.S., there is no universal right to health, to health care services, or even to insurance coverage of health care expenses. This sets the U.S. apart from every other highly developed nation, and from some less-developed countries, as well. The key distinction is that in this country we generally treat access to health services like we treat access to food, shelter, automobiles, and vacuum cleaners, which is to say you are welcome to them if you can afford them; in other developed countries, there is a sense that basic human rights standards include a distinct right to health care services. In the former instance health care services are viewed as a commodity, whereas in the latter case health care is seen as a public good worthy of promoting through wealth redistribution.

The choice to commodify health care services—and therefore exclude tens of millions of people from being able to afford it—comes with significant costs to society, and many of the more obvious costs are discussed at points throughout this text. At the same time, there are less obvious ways in which our for-profit health care system harms people. For example, one consequence of the nation's failure to grant equal access to health care services is to actually make people *feel* excluded. Indeed, access to health insurance and health care services functions as a type of social institution, in that having access to these goods shapes behaviors, offers the potential for upward mobility, and fosters feelings of belonging and dignity. The reverse is also true: "In addition to the stress, powerlessness and social disrespect that have been shown to be associated with poorer health status, [uninsured individuals'] awareness of their disadvantaged social status has the potential to undermine self-respect and their sense of themselves as the moral equals of the more fortunate members of society."[6] Furthermore, "where state and local governments have made a concerted effort to integrate marginalized populations into the health care system, researchers find greater connectedness, collaboration, and feelings of a shared fate."[7]

▶ The Role of Social Determinants in Individual and Population Health

According to the U.S. Department of Health and Human Services, social determinants of health are those "[c]onditions in the environments in which people are born, live, learn, work, play, worship, and age that affect a wide range of health, functioning, and quality-of-life outcomes and risks."[8] There are many examples of these types of social factors—neighborhood conditions (including the amount of crime and violence), housing quality, early childhood education and development, economic stability, access to transportation, employment, access to sufficient amounts of healthy food, access to health care services, a community's level of social cohesion— and they are key drivers of health inequalities, health disparities, and health care disparities. Sadly, the overall level of health inequality has been on the rise in the U.S.

over the past several decades and is now among the highest in developed countries as measured by differences in life expectancy, the number of people who are uninsured, the amount of money that individuals spend on health care needs relative to their overall income, and the level of racial and ethnic health disparities.

One immediate takeaway for readers is that the conditions in which people live, work, and play have an enormous impact on individual (and thus community) health totally irrespective of whether a person ever sees the inside of a doctor's office. To better understand this, let's zero in on differences in life expectancy, one of the metrics noted above that is used to comparatively measure health inequality. At time of birth, life expectancy in the U.S. can vary by as many as 25 years depending on the location in which a person is born. For example, the next baby to be born in Eagle County, Colorado (one of the counties with the highest life expectancy in the U.S.) has an average life expectancy that is more than two decades longer than the next baby to be born in Ogala Lakota County, South Dakota (a county near the bottom in terms of life expectancy). You can drive from one county to the other in about 8 hours. Even starker, perhaps, is an example from Philadelphia, Pennsylvania. A child born today in the area covered by the 19106 zip code—near the Delaware River and the famed Liberty Bell—has a life expectancy of 88 years. Less than four miles away in the area covered by the 19132 zip code, a child's life expectancy at birth is just 68 years. That 20-year difference represents approximately one year for each minute it takes to drive between the two locations. In these examples you get a sense of why social and environmental factors are bigger drivers of health than either genes or access to health care services: no amount of good genes or doctor visits could ever correct these differences in life expectancy, but realigning social factors that influence health could dramatically level the playing field. In fact, the concept of "luck egalitarianism"—the idea that justice requires correcting disadvantages resulting from brute luck—has gained ground in recent years, including in the context of health and health care.[9] If society did more correcting of this type, we would reduce differences in the key determinants of health, in turn reducing health inequalities and disparities, and thus move closer to achieving health justice.

▶ Wealth Equals Health

Closely related to the discussion about social determinants of health is the fact that generally speaking, a person or community's wealth effectively determines that person or community's overall level of health; in turn, one's level of health affects one's ability to improve upon his or her economic status, since it is exceedingly difficult to overcome the forces associated with low economic status without good health. Consider the following:

- Over the last 30 years, life expectancy has increased dramatically among people in the top half of the income distribution, while remaining close to flat among those in the bottom half.[10]
- The risk of dying before the age of 65 is more than three times greater for those with low socioeconomic status (SES) than for those with high SES.[11]
- Almost every chronic condition, including stroke, heart disease, and arthritis, follows a predictable pattern: prevalence increases as income decreases.[12]
- People living in poverty are disproportionately burdened by the communal consequences of poor health: higher crime rates, decreased residential home values, and higher health care costs.[13]

- Poor and middle-class individuals pay a larger share of their incomes for health care than do the affluent, thereby deepening inequalities in disposable income.[14]
- Because health care indebtedness is the single largest cause of personal bankruptcy, many low-income individuals forego needed health care rather than risk indebtedness.

Taken together, the literature on the connection between wealth and health provides "overwhelming evidence that economically disadvantaged groups have poorer survival chances and a higher mortality rate, die at a younger age, experience a blighted quality of life, and have overall diminished health and well-being when compared to other members of society."[15] This wealth-health connection links back to the previous two overarching topics: the nation's treatment of health care as a commodity makes it more difficult for people stuck on the lower rungs of the SES ladder to achieve good health, and economic deprivation is a type of social determinant that would require purposeful correction if health justice is to be achieved. Indeed, it is widely known and accepted that income inequality in the U.S. is greater than in any other developed nation, has been growing for decades, and currently rests at historically high levels, with the top 1% of earners taking home nearly a quarter of the nation's income.

▶ Society Medicalizes Social Needs and Criminalizes Social Deficiencies

The final topic we introduce here to contextualize the concept of health justice focuses on the ways in which the nation underappreciates and misconstrues the role played by social supports in the overall health of the population. To begin, review **FIGURE 1**.

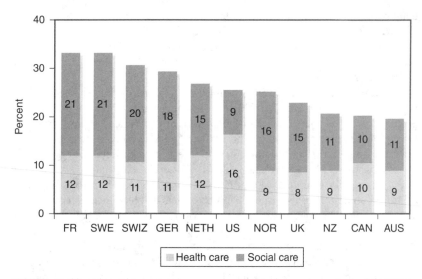

FIGURE 1 Health and social care spending as a percentage of gross domestic product (GDP).

Reproduced from The Brookings Institute. Health and Social Care Spending as a Percentage of GDP. Retreived from: https://www
.brookings.edu/blog/up-front/2017/02/15/re-balancing-medical-and-social-spending-to-promote-health-increasing-state-flexibility
-to-improve-health-through-housing.

Note how, as a percentage of gross domestic product (GDP), combined U.S. spending on health and social care sits right in the middle of the pack when compared to some other developed nations. But the real story resides in how the country spends that money: unlike every other nation represented, the U.S. spends more money on health care than on social care (services targeting education, housing, nutrition, poverty, and the like), and it spends less money on social care (as a percentage of GDP) than every other nation.[16] Given these spending patterns, you might think that while we spend less than perhaps we should on social care, our runaway spending on health care would keep us fairly healthy as a nation. Unfortunately, this is far from the case. Compared to most other developed countries, the U.S. actually has similar or worse outcomes on several key measures of health, including maternal health, infant mortality, and chronic disease prevention. What is likely occurring is that instead of spending money on supports and programs that could keep people healthy (or healthier) in the first instance, the nation is overspending on relatively expensive medical treatments and procedures once individuals become ill,[17] then sending people back into communities that lack sufficient social supports, thus starting the cycle over again. This is what we mean when we say that the U.S. "medicalizes" social needs: essentially, health care services are compensating for a lack of social services spending.

In addition to medicalizing social needs, our society too often criminalizes social deficiencies. Let's use the lack of affordable housing as the first example of a social deficiency. The demand for affordable housing is immense, as very low-income earners represent 24% of all renter households and 9% of all U.S. households. Yet according to multiple reports, there is not a single county in the U.S. that can fill 100% of its low-income population's need for safe, affordable housing[18] and, on average, there are only 35 adequate and affordable housing options for every 100 very low-income households nationally. Making matters worse: the poorer the household, the worse the situation, as families with incomes in the bottom 15% of all earners face the prospect of just 17 affordable units available per 100 households. Two root causes of these deficiencies include a lack of investment in affordable housing development and generally relentless rent inflation, which usually hits the lowest-income earners the hardest.

The lack of affordable housing—coupled with the lack of available shelter space, which represents another social deficiency—subjugates hundreds of thousands of people to a life on the streets. Being homeless, in turn, often prompts responses from police, particularly as states and localities pass laws and ordinances making it a crime to perform life-sustaining activities (e.g., eating, sleeping, begging, etc.) in public spaces. These interactions can have terrible consequences for people already struggling to survive, as some homeless people have their personal property destroyed, some are pushed out of the urban centers that tend to have more reliable social supports, some accumulate fines they can't afford to pay, and many develop criminal records, which makes it more difficult to secure employment or housing. Additionally, many homeless persons who come into contact with police are temporarily incarcerated, which standing alone can be devastating: research indicates that being incarcerated for even just a few days can adversely impact future chances of employment and the well-being of dependent children. It is worth noting that incarcerating homeless persons costs two to three times as much as providing long-term supportive housing.[19]

A second example—this one related to the nation's mental health and substance use crises—drives home the point about how society too easily criminalizes social deficiencies. To start, it is important to understand that compared against every other nation in the world, the U.S. has the highest incarceration rate: approximately 700 people for every 100,000 residents are in jails or prisons.[20] No other country has a rate that tops 600 people per 100,000 residents, and save for a handful of nations, all countries are below 400 people per 100,000 residents.[21] The median rate is approximately 150 prisoners per 100,000 residents. Another way to understand the nation's incarceration rate is to grasp that while the U.S. has only 5% of the world's population, it has nearly 25% of its prisoners—which equates to 2.2 million people on any given day. (It must also be noted that U.S. prisons and jails are disproportionately populated with members of racial and ethnic minority groups. For example, while people of color make up just over 30% of the general population, they comprise more than half of the jail/prison population.[22] While blacks make up approximately 13% of the nation's population, they account for 28% of all arrests, 40% of the incarcerated population, and 42% of the population on death row.[23] And Native Americans are incarcerated at more than twice the rate of whites, while Latinos are held under state jurisdiction at 1.7 times the rate for whites.[24]) Emerging research indicates that this level of mass incarceration may be harming entire communities and contributing to health disparities in the U.S.[25]

A few of the things that drive the U.S. incarceration rate do, in fact, have more to do with criminal justice policy and less about social care deficiencies. For example, the move to mandatory minimum sentences and the implementation of tough-on-crime policies—including "three-strikes" laws and requirements that prisoners serve at least 85% of their sentences—help keep prisons well stocked. But another significant driver of the incarceration rate is society's unwillingness to grapple with its mental health and substance use crises. Some 64% of jail inmates, 54% of state prisoners, and 45% of federal prisoners report mental health concerns, and studies have shown that 65% of jail inmates meet standards for a diagnosable substance abuse disorder.[26] Overall, approximately 79% of prisoners suffer from either drug addiction or mental illness, and 40% suffer from both.[27] Indeed, the number of individuals with serious mental illness in prisons and jails now exceeds by ten times the number in state psychiatric hospitals, and there are more people behind bars for a drug offense than the number of people who were in prison or jail for *any* crime in 1980.[28] Essentially, prisons and jails have become a stand-in for treatment clinics and rehabilitation facilities. Rather than provide prevention, treatment, and other supports in the first instance to individuals who suffer from treatable mental health and substance use disorders, society defaults to the more dangerous, less-effective, and more expensive option—criminalizing the behavior that often results from illness.

▶ Rationale for and Structure of *Essentials of Health Justice: A Primer*

In recent years, greater attention on the part of policymakers, health professionals, and educators to health disparities and to the social determinants of health has led to more inclusion of these topics in public health, medicine, nursing, health care administration, social work, and law curricula. Indeed, either as a standalone elective course or as a component of a required course, health equity is now a fairly common topic in public health and other health professions education, and beginning in December 2018, the topics of law, policy, and health equity/social justice will together make up 30% of the content used to certify public health professionals in the examination given by the National Board of Public Health Examiners.

Essentials of Health Justice: A Primer was designed with this evolution in mind, and can be used as a standalone text or as a supplement to a wide range of public health, health administration, medicine, nursing, health policy, and health law textbooks. Created as an interdisciplinary teaching tool, it explores how health and justice intersect, how law and policy shape the health care and public health systems and the social structures affecting health outcomes, how disparate impacts of these structures affect particular populations, how social and medical systems may be reshaped to be more responsive to health inequity, and how individuals can advocate for systems change and health justice. Furthermore, this text aims to connect population health and well-being with general education and the Association of American Colleges and Universities' focus on social justice (www.aacu.org/making-excellence-inclusive).

Essentials of Health Justice: A Primer is divided into three parts. Part I is titled "Context and Background: Health-Harming Legal Doctrines, Historical Discrimination, and Implicit Bias" and includes chapters on health-harming legal doctrines (Chapter 1) and the health effects of explicit discrimination and implicit bias (Chapter 2). Part II, titled "Health Disparities and Their Structural Underpinnings" more fully describes the myriad health disparities that affect various populations (Chapter 3) and delineates the pathological social structures and systems that lead to and perpetuate health inequity (Chapter 4). Part III turns its attention to "Striving for Health Justice" by describing existing safety net programs and some health-related legal protections in the U.S. (Chapter 5), the types of coordinated systems that are needed to care for socially complex patients and populations (Chapter 6), and the ways in which readers of this text can advocate for health justice (Chapter 7). The text concludes with a call to action to recognize and affirm that the lives of medically and socially vulnerable populations can be immeasurably improved by respecting those populations' right to health justice.

References

1. Braveman P, Arkin E, Orleans T, Proctor D, Plough A. *What Is Health Equity? And What Difference Does a Definition Make?* Brooklyn, NY: Robert Wood Johnson Foundation; 2017. Available at: http://www.buildhealthyplaces.org/content/uploads/2017/05/rwjf436997.pdf.
2. World Health Organization. Health Impact Assessment Programme: glossary of terms used. Available at: http://www.who.int/hia/about/glos/en/index1.html.
3. Woolf S. Progress in achieving health equity requires attention to root causes. *Health Affairs.* June 2017;36(6):984–991.
4. U.S. Department of Health and Human Services. The Secretary's Advisory Committee on National Health Promotion and Disease Prevention Objectives for 2020. Phase I report: recommendations for the framework and format of Healthy People 2020; 2008. Section IV: Advisory Committee findings and recommendations. Available at: http://www.healthypeople.gov/sites/default/files/PhaseI_0.pdf.
5. Smedley B, Stith A, Nelson A, eds. Unequal treatment: confronting racial and ethnic disparities in health care. Washington, DC: Institute of Medicine; 2003. Available at: http://www.nap.edu/openbook.php?isbn=030908265X.
6. Faden R, Powers M. Incrementalism: ethical implications of policy choices. The Kaiser Family Foundation; 1999. Available at: https://kaiserfamilyfoundation.files.wordpress.com/2013/01/incrementalism-ethical-implications-of-policy-choices-issue-paper.pdf.

7. McKay T. The social costs of repealing the ACA. *Health Affairs* blog; March 7, 2017. Available at: http://healthaffairs.org/blog/2017/03/07/the-social-costs-of-repealing-the-aca-2/.

8. U.S. Department of Health and Human Services. The Secretary's Advisory Committee on National Health Promotion and Disease Prevention Objectives. 2020 topics and objectives: social determinants of health. Available at: https://www.healthypeople.gov/2020/topics-objectives/topic/social-determinants-of-health.

9. Segall S. *Health, Luck, and Justice.* Princeton, NJ: Princeton University Press; 2009.

10. Wiley L. Health law as social justice. *Cornell Journal of Law and Public Policy.* 2014;24(1):47.

11. Benfer EA. Health justice: a framework (and call to action) for the elimination of health inequity and social justice. *American University Law Review.* 2015;65(2):278–279.

12. Dickman SL, Himmelstein DU, Woolhandler S. Inequality and the health-care system in the USA. *Lancet.* 2017;389:1431–1444.

13. Benfer EA. Health justice: a framework (and call to action) for the elimination of health inequity and social justice. *American University Law Review.* 2015;65(2):278–279.

14. Dickman SL, Himmelstein DU, Woolhandler S. Inequality and the health-care system in the USA. *Lancet.* 2017;389:1431–1444.

15. Benfer EA. Health justice: a framework (and call to action) for the elimination of health inequity and social justice. *American University Law Review.* 2015;65(2):278–279.

16. Brookings Institution. Health and social care spending as a percentage of gross domestic product (GDP); 2017. Available at: https://www.brookings.edu/blog/up-front/2017/02/15/re-balancing-medical-and-social-spending-to-promote-health-increasing-state-flexibility-to-improve-health-through-housing.

17. Butler SM. Social spending, not medical spending, is key to health. Brookings Institution; 2016. Available at: https://www.brookings.edu/opinions/social-spending-not-medical-spending-is-key-to-health/; Bradley EH, Taylor LA. How social spending affects health outcomes. Robert Wood Johnson Foundation; 2016. Available at: http://www.rwjf.org/en/culture-of-health/2016/08/how_social_spending.html.

18. Aurand A, Emmanuel D, Yentel D, Errico E. *The Gap: A Shortage of Affordable Homes.* The National Low Income Housing Coalition; March 2017. Available at: http://nlihc.org/research/gap-report; Leopold J, Getsinger L, Blumenthal P, Abazajian K, Jordan R. The housing affordability gap for extremely low-income renters in 2013. The Urban Institute; June 2015. Available at: http://www.urban.org/research/publication/housing-affordability-gap-extremely-low-income-renters-2013/view/full_report.

19. Hodge, Jr. J, DiPietro B, Horton-Newell AE. Homelessness and the public's health: legal responses. *Journal of Law, Medicine & Ethics.* 2017;45(1):28–32.

20. Wagner P, Walsh A. States of incarceration: the global context 2016. Prison Policy Initiative; June 16, 2016. Available at: https://www.prisonpolicy.org/global/2016.html.

21. *Id.*

22. National Association for the Advancement of Colored People (NAACP). Criminal justice fact sheet. Available at: http://www.naacp.org/criminal-justice-fact-sheet/.

23. Hartney C, Vuong L. Created equal: racial and ethnic disparities in the U.S. criminal justice system. National Council on Crime and Delinquency; 2009. Available at: http://www.nccdglobal.org/sites/default/files/publication_pdf/created-equal.pdf.

24. *Id.*

25. Wildeman C, Wang E. Mass incarceration, public health, and widening inequality in the USA. *Lancet.* 2017;389:1464–1474.

26. American Psychological Association (APA). Incarceration Nation; 2014. Available at: http://www.apa.org/monitor/2014/10/incarceration.aspx.

27. Austin J, Eisen LB, Cullen J, Frank J. How many Americans are unnecessarily incarcerated? Brennan Center for Justice, NYU School of Law; 2016. Available at: https://www.brennancenter.org/sites/default/files/publications/Unnecessarily_Incarcerated_0.pdf.

28. The Sentencing Project. Criminal justice facts. Available at: http://www.sentencingproject.org/criminal-justice-facts/.

Context and Background: Health-Harming Legal Doctrines, Historical Discrimination, and Implicit Bias

Part I of this text includes two chapters aimed at introducing readers to relevant legal doctrines and to the lasting health effects of the nation's discriminatory past. By way of background, Chapter 1 describes four different health-harming legal doctrines. Chapter 2 discusses the health-related legacy of race-based discrimination and the ongoing effects of implicit bias on health and health care.

Health-Harming Legal Doctrines

▶ Introduction

This chapter provides readers with an overview of the types of broad legal doctrines that can influence the health of tens of millions of people—even when the doctrines themselves have nothing specific to do with health or health care. We start here because it represents one of the broadest possible ways to begin a discussion about health justice: by zooming out to consider the topic through a very wide lens, so that from the outset readers understand that even arcane legal doctrines seemingly unrelated to health equity are at work to influence the nation's health in disproportionate ways. As the text progresses, the lens zooms in more and more, providing a series of images that portray health injustices in sharper relief.

We've selected four legal doctrines to serve as examples, a couple of which receive additional treatment in subsequent chapters. The selected doctrines were not chosen for their interrelatedness; indeed, in some cases, they have little to do with one another, aside from the fact that they all work in their own way to make it more difficult for many people to get and/or stay healthy. The first doctrine discussed was alluded to in the Introduction to this text, and it is the only one of the four that is specific to health care services: the "no duty to treat" principle. This long-standing principle helps explain why there is no overarching right to health care in the United States, and is a natural starting point for a discussion about health justice. The second doctrine has to do with the fact that federal civil rights protections have never been extended to poverty in the same way they have been extended to race, ethnicity, gender, disability, age, and other traits or distinguishing qualities. We next discuss the notion of a "negative Constitution," which refers to the fact that the federal Constitution has been interpreted by the U.S. Supreme Court as not *requiring* the government to affirmatively act to protect the public's health and welfare. Lastly, we explain the difference between the right to legal counsel in criminal matters and in civil legal matters. The lack of such a right in the latter context can have enormous health consequences for low-income individuals and families.

▶ The "No Duty to Treat" Principle

One of the most basic tenets in U.S. health law is that generally speaking, individuals have no legal right to health care services (or to health insurance). As a result, there is no legal responsibility on the part of clinicians to provide health care upon request. This doctrine is referred to as the "no duty" or "no duty to treat" principle, which is perhaps most famously described in the case of *Hurley v. Eddingfield*. In that case, the Indiana Supreme Court was asked to pass judgment on the actions of one Dr. Eddingfield, whose lack of medical attention led to the death of a pregnant woman named Charlotte Burk. In the course of discussing whether the doctor had a legal relationship to Mrs. Burk sufficient to trigger a duty to treat, the court wrote that Indiana's medical licensing statute:

> provides for . . . standards of qualification . . . and penalties for practicing without a license. The [state licensing] act is preventive, not a compulsive, measure. In obtaining the state's license (permission) to practice medicine, the state does not require, and the licensee does not engage, that he will practice at all or on other terms than he may choose to accept.[1]

In other words, according to the court, Dr. Eddingfield's medical license did not confer upon him an *obligation* to provide health care services; rather, Indiana's licensure requirement existed in order to make sure that should a person actually decide to provide health care services, that person would have the necessary knowledge and skills to do so in an appropriate fashion. Viewed in this way, medical licenses are a form of quality control, not a mechanism for gaining access to services. The same can be said for the driver's licenses many of you have in your book bag or purse: in no way does it require that you take a vehicle out for a spin, today or ever; rather, as with a medical license, the point of your driver's license is to guarantee that should you *choose* to operate a motor vehicle, you are qualified to do so. Note too that just as Dr. Eddingfield's medical license did not grant Mrs. Burk access to his services, your driver's license does not grant you access to a car or truck.

In order to understand the power of the "no duty" principle, you should know one other thing about Dr. Eddingfield: prior to Charlotte Burk's death, he served as her family physician. Put in more formal terms, the doctor had a preexisting relationship with the now-deceased patient. Clearly the Indiana Supreme Court was aware of this fact from the record that was produced during the doctor's trial, and surely, you must be thinking, this fact would establish enough of a fiduciary relationship to hold Dr. Eddingfield accountable for the death of Mrs. Burk. However, under the law, physician–patient relationships must be established (and re-established) for each specific "spell of illness," and thus past treatment alone is not enough to form a legally binding relationship in the present. Put differently, a physician–patient relationship does not exist as a general, continuous legal matter—even with one's primary care doctor—but rather it exists for a specific period of time and must be (re)established accordingly.

As noted in the Introduction to this text, the U.S. generally treats health care as a commodity subject to market forces and to one's own economic status. Indeed, during the public debate in 1993 over President William Clinton's failed attempt at national health reform—one of several times the nation has debated whether to move away from the "no duty" principle and establish a right to health care—then–U.S. Representative Dick Armey (R-TX) stated that "health care is just a commodity, just like bread, and just like housing and everything else."[2] What is instructive about Representative Armey's quote is that, far from being a legal anomaly, the lack of a right to health care services is in line with the nation's overall approach to access to basic necessities. During the 1960s and early 1970s, with the tailwinds of the Civil Rights Movement filling their sails, a determined group of public interest lawyers and social reform activists pressed the federal courts for an interpretation of the Constitution that would have created an individual right to welfare. Under this view, the government would be required to provide individuals who suffered from "brutal need" with minimally adequate levels of health care, food, housing, etc.—the types of things referred to by Representative Armey. But in a series of cases, the Supreme Court rejected this notion of a constitutional right to welfare. Underpinning these decisions were views about the nature and design of the Constitution, the nation's free market philosophies, and more.

At the same time, the scope of the "no duty to treat" principle is not all-encompassing, as there are a few laws that chip away at it and thus carve out a right to health care services where otherwise it would not exist. For example, a federal law called the *Examination and Treatment for Emergency Medical Conditions and Women in Labor Act* grants all individuals, irrespective of one's ability to pay or a hospital's willingness to provide services, the right to an "appropriate screening examination" and, if an emergency condition is uncovered, to clinical services necessary to stabilize the patient. Basically, the law prevents hospitals from turning away people with medical emergencies—at least until those emergencies have been addressed to the point that the individual's condition will not materially worsen upon leaving the facility, at which time the "no duty" principle kicks back in and the hospital is free to refuse further treatment. Additionally, both Medicaid and Medicare create legal rights to health care benefits and services for individuals who meet the programs' eligibility criteria, but then again, these services are only carried out by health care providers who choose in the first instance to participate in the programs themselves. (Recall the analogy between a medical license and a driver's license; in the case of providers who choose not to participate in Medicaid and Medicare, they are effectively choosing the types of cars they don't want to drive.) Finally, some private health insurance products obligate physicians participating in the delivery of those products to provide care to individuals who purchase those products; essentially, for purposes of this discussion, delivery of care under these private health insurance policies operates like the delivery of Medicaid and Medicare services, in the sense that physicians decide whether to become "participating providers" in private health insurance plans.

The basic upshot of the "no duty" principle is that individuals can access health care services if (1) they have the means to pay for health care services outright; (2) they have the means to pay for private health insurance premiums, deductibles, and copayments; (3) they have been singled out for public insurance coverage on the basis of medical condition, age, or income; or (4) they are lucky enough to stumble into free services through the magnanimity of ethics-conscious health care providers. It almost goes without saying that this approach to health care results in enormous gaps: as discussed in the chapter on health disparities, the nation suffers from disparities in health care access, diagnosis, treatment, and outcomes, based on a range of factors including race, ethnicity, socioeconomic status, physical and mental disability, age, gender, sexual orientation, and immigration status. Furthermore, it is common for people to forego care altogether on the basis of cost. Recent data indicate that 55% of people without insurance coverage, 30% of people with private insurance, and 21% of people with public insurance said they had forgone needed health care because it was too expensive.[3]

▸ The Exclusion of Poverty from Protection Under the Constitution

In the chapter on social and structural barriers to health, you will learn about the close connection between poverty and poor health. As a backdrop to that discussion, we describe here the way in which poverty has been treated under the federal Constitution—namely, as underserving of rigorous antidiscrimination protection. Certain characteristics such as race, ethnicity, national origin, religion, and gender have been declared "suspect" or "quasi-suspect" classes by the U.S. Supreme Court, a designation that indicates that people have suffered governmental discrimination on the basis of these characteristics in the past. As a result, the Court has interpreted the federal Constitution's Equal Protection Clause in a way that grants special protection against discrimination to these classes. However, the Court has never ruled that the impoverished are a protected class. Furthermore, the Court has protected over time certain fundamental rights—including rights not explicitly set out in the Constitution—under the Constitution's Due Process Clause. Notwithstanding a series of cases the Court heard during the Civil Rights Era, the Court has yet to find that individuals have a fundamental right to even the most basic necessities.

Overview of Equal Protection Jurisprudence

Under the Equal Protection Clause of the Fourteenth Amendment to the federal Constitution, states are generally prohibited from governing in ways that single out particular groups for unequal treatment.[4] Nonetheless, a state will often pass laws that treat certain groups differently than others, such as a law that prohibits men—but not women—under a certain age from purchasing alcohol.[5] As described below, whether this law (and many others that similarly differentiate among groups of people, regardless of the context) is constitutional depends in large part upon how deeply a court scrutinizes a legislature's goals in passing the law. The important idea that there should be different levels of judicial scrutiny when undertaking equal protection analyses was born in a surprising place: a footnote in a 1938 Supreme Court decision considering a state law concerning milk. In discussing the Court's practice to normally defer to states about their reasons for passing laws, Justice Harlan Stone recognized that, in contrast to economic laws like the one before the Court, "prejudice against discrete and insular minorities may be a special condition, which tends seriously to curtail the operation of those political processes ordinarily to be relied upon to protect minorities, and which may call for a correspondingly more searching judicial inquiry."[6] In other words, when legislatures pass laws that disadvantage "discrete and insular minorities," the lawmakers may have been motivated not by neutral governmental goals like safety, but rather by prejudice or animus. As a result, courts should be in the habit of carefully scrutinizing those laws that may have been corrupted by hostility towards certain minority groups.

One question the Court has had to answer several times since 1938 is: which groups are "discrete and insular minorities"? Although the Court has not ruled that any particular set of criteria must be satisfied in order to qualify a group as a "suspect class," it has generally asked at least three questions when considering this question:

1. Has the group in question historically been discriminated against or been subject to prejudice, hostility, or stigma?
2. Does the group possess an immutable or highly visible trait?
3. Is the group generally powerless to protect itself through the political process?

Only a few years after writing its famous footnote, the Supreme Court determined that laws "which curtail the civil rights of a single racial group are immediately suspect" and as a result, the Court will apply "the most rigid scrutiny" when deciding their constitutionality.[7] Under this "strict scrutiny" test, as it has come to be known, race-based classifications will be upheld only if the law has a compelling government interest and is narrowly tailored to achieving it. Strict scrutiny has proven to be a difficult standard to overcome, because it is very hard for a state legislature to show that a law favoring one race over another has a compelling governmental objective behind it. The Court now also applies strict scrutiny to laws treating U.S. citizens differently than noncitizens, laws singling out individuals based on their national origin, and laws infringing fundamental rights.

Through the process of deciding which groups are worthy of enhanced protection from discrimination, the Supreme Court determined that laws that treat men and women differently are not as plainly troubling as classifications based on race, national origin, or citizenship status. As a result, the Court deemed sex-based laws "quasi-suspect," subjecting them not to strict but to "intermediate" scrutiny. Under this standard, states must show that a law that classifies people on the basis of sex serves important governmental objectives and is substantially related to the achievement of those objectives.[8]

Applying a variety of factors, with varying degrees of consistency, the Court has found that not all groups singled out for disparate treatment should be subjected to strict or even intermediate scrutiny.[9] If the Court determines that the classification is neither suspect nor quasi-suspect, it applies the lowest standard of review, termed "rational basis" review. Laws nearly always survive this type of review. For example, the Supreme Court upheld a Massachusetts law that required police officers to retire at age 50, refusing to find that age was a suspect or quasi-suspect classification, citing no history of discrimination and the fact that older people cannot be a discrete, insular minority because everyone ages. The Court scrutinized the law only to the extent of asking whether the law was rationally related to a legitimate state inter-est, and was satisfied with testimony that, because people tend to decline physically at age 50, the law serves the state's interest in public safety.[10] However, even when applying rational basis review, the Court will refuse to uphold a law if it is based upon "a bare ... desire to harm a politically unpopular group."[11]

Overview of Substantive Due Process Jurisprudence

Just as the Fourteenth Amendment limits the ability of governments to single out particular groups for unequal treatment, it also protects individuals from laws that infringe too severely upon fundamental rights guaranteed by the Constitution. This is known as the guarantee to "substantive due process," because the protections stem from the Fourteenth Amendment's Due Process Clause. Some fundamental rights, like the right to vote, are explicitly included in the text of the Constitution. Others, however, are not explicitly mentioned but are so "deeply rooted in the Nation's history and tradition" and "implicit in the concept of ordered liberty" that the Supreme Court has deemed them to be fundamental (for example, rights related to marriage, contraception, procreation, and child rearing).

As with determining which suspect or quasi-suspect groups fall under the Equal Protection umbrella, the Court has grappled with determining which implicit rights are worthy of being classified as fundamental. In what is clearly the most famous example, the Court found in *Roe v. Wade* that the fundamental (but implicit) right to privacy was expansive enough to encompass a woman's right to choose to terminate a pregnancy under certain circumstances.[12]

Efforts to Apply Equal Protection and Substantive Due Process to Laws Affecting the Poor

Concurrent with other social movements of the time, the 1960s and early 1970s brought about a fight for equality for poor people, as advocates sought to publicize the harms associated with persistent poverty, poor nutrition, dangerous housing, and substandard education. And while the federal Aid to Families with Dependent Children (AFDC) program (which started in 1935 as a relatively minor expendi-ture but became a nearly $30 billion program by the mid-1970s) provided assistance for struggling families, the often humiliating and burdensome legal requirements imposed by states in administering it solidified the general view that recipients were second-class citizens.[13] Poverty lawyers launched challenges to these state laws on various grounds, including the argument that they infringed upon an implicit fun-damental right: the right to live at a basic level of subsistence.

The first state welfare law challenge that made its way to the U.S. Supreme Court, in a case called *King v. Smith*, was successful—just not on constitutional grounds. In the *King* case, the state of Alabama terminated welfare benefits to a single mother because she occasionally cohabitated with a man who was not her husband, on the grounds that this man acted as a "substitute father" and could sup-port the woman's children. The Supreme Court rejected this argument, finding it to be a violation of the federal AFDC statute, which only denied benefits where legal parents—but not men who cohabitate with single mothers—were able to provide support.[14] *King v. Smith* marked a victory for the welfare rights movement, but it did nothing to improve efforts to gain special status for the poor under the Constitution.

The second welfare benefits case to be heard by the Court, *Shapiro v. Thompson*, challenged a Connecticut rule that denied welfare benefits to families that had lived in the state for less than a year. This time, the Court decided the case on constitutional grounds, holding that the rule infringed on the plaintiff's implicit fundamental right to travel and could not survive strict scrutiny.[15] Even though the Court held that the law infringed upon the right to travel, and not on a right to live, the decision resulted in a "euphoric reception from welfare lawyers," who hoped "that strict scrutiny would soon be extended to state welfare law classifications, heralding the end of geographic differences in welfare grants and moving inexorably toward a constitutional right to live."[16]

Soon after, in 1970, poverty lawyers recorded another victory in *Goldberg v. Kelly*, when the Court held that welfare benefits could not be terminated without an evidentiary hearing. Importantly, the Court considered the welfare benefits to be "statutory entitlements" rather than charity, but it did not go so far as to find that the poor have a constitutional right to receive welfare benefits.[17] Nevertheless, the Court noted that:

> …important governmental interests are promoted by affording recipients a pre-termination evidentiary hearing. From its founding, the Nation's basic commitment has been to foster the dignity and wellbeing of all persons within its borders. We have come to recognize that forces not within the control of the poor contribute to their poverty…Welfare, by meeting the basic demands of subsistence, can help bring within the reach of the poor the same opportunities that are available to others to participate meaningfully in the life of the community… Public assistance, then, is not mere charity, but a means to 'promote the general Welfare, and secure the Blessings of Liberty to ourselves and our Posterity.' The same governmental interests that counsel the provision of welfare, counsel as well its uninterrupted provision to those eligible to receive it; pre-termination evidentiary hearings are indispensable to that end.[18]

The Court's strong language—and its quotation of the Preamble to the Constitution—suggested to some that the Court was sloping toward a future ruling that those mired in poverty had a right to public assistance, thus taking another step closer to recognizing a right to live.

However, the Court abruptly halted this trajectory in *Dandridge v. Williams*, decided just a few weeks after *Goldberg*. The issue in *Dandridge* was whether a Maryland regulation setting a family maximum limit for welfare benefits violated the Equal Protection Clause because it unfairly disadvantaged families with more children by providing less money per child. The Court was blunt in its assessment, characterizing state welfare rules as the type of "intractable economic, social and even philosophical problems" that are "not the business of this Court." Applying the lowest level of scrutiny, the Court upheld the law as rationally related to the state's legitimate interests, including encouraging employment.[19]

In another case arguing for special legal status for poor people, called *San Antonio Independent School District v. Rodriguez*, students in a poor area of San Antonio challenged Texas' method of funding public education. The method, wherein school districts in relatively wealthy areas provided more funding per student than did districts with poorer residents, was challenged under the Equal Protection Clause for providing lower quality education to poor children. In response, the Supreme Court refused to find that children living in poorer school districts were entitled to a public education equal to that of children from wealthier families, noting that it had never found that wealth is a suspect class entitled to strict scrutiny.[20] The Court wrote that "at least where wealth is involved, the Equal Protection Clause does not require absolute equality or precisely equal advantages." The Court contrasted this case to earlier decisions, in which wealth-based classifications completely deprived individuals of important services and were struck down as a result. As a result, the Court applied rational basis review and affirmed Texas' funding scheme.

Future Prospects for Granting Poverty Special Status

The line of welfare rights cases culminating in *Dandridge* seems to foreclose a finding that there is a fundamental right to live, a right for which many poverty lawyers had fought.[21] But the Court's language in *Goldberg* at least suggests a way forward for future arguments that a person mired in poverty has a right to a basic level of subsistence. Since public assistance, in the form of welfare, subsidized housing, subsidized nutrition, a quality education, and more, is needed to sustain even a meager existence for millions of adults and kids, perhaps society should consider whether a legally recognized, even if implicit, fundamental right to live should be "found" in the nation's Constitution.[22]

Furthermore, although the Supreme Court in *Rodriguez* was stating the obvious when it said it has never held that poverty is a suspect class, this is primarily a product of the Court's unwillingness to address the question directly.[23] Were the Court to consider the standards under which other classifications have been deemed suspect, it could certainly find that laws singling out the poor should be more closely scrutinized. As the state welfare laws above demonstrate, there is a long history of discrimination against the poor. Further, there can be no doubt that low-income individuals lack political power, given that ordinary political processes are often dominated by corporate interests and wealthy individuals.[24] At the very least, laws which discriminate against the poor and are rooted in "a bare ... desire to harm a politically unpopular group" should be subjected to more searching review.[25]

▶ The "Negative Constitution"

We turn now to a third health-harming legal doctrine, this one termed the "negative Constitution." This discussion certainly dovetails with the one immediately above, since the negative Constitution helps to explain why certain positive rights (like rights to tangible things, including food or health care services) are not often found to exist as a federal constitutional matter.

By way of background, we start with a description of what are known as "police powers." These powers represent state and local government authority to require conformance with certain standards of conduct meant to protect the public's health, safety, and welfare. Put less formally, a state's police powers allow it to control—to some extent—personal and corporate activities that may harm the public's health if left unbridled. There are many examples of police powers: health care providers must obtain licenses from state agencies before practicing medicine; health care facilities must meet and maintain certain accreditation standards; restaurants are heavily regulated by states and localities; employers must follow many occupational health and safety rules, and buildings have "codes" that must be followed when they are designed, built, and maintained; certain industries are constrained by pollution control measures; the marketing and sale of tobacco products is regulated by law; motorcyclists must wear helmets, passengers in cars must wear seat belts. If you stopped to think about it for a couple minutes, you would likely generate many more examples of the ways in which your daily activities are shaped by governmental police powers.

As the above list indicates, police powers can be rather coercive, if not downright invasive. However, these powers are not absolute, and at some point they give way to the individual freedoms and liberties we have come to cherish as Americans. Furthermore, police powers can never be used to purely punish individuals—since their purpose is the promotion of public health—they cannot be administered arbitrarily, and they cannot be used for purposes unrelated to public welfare.

After reading about police powers, many students reasonably believe that states *must* protect the public health and welfare through affirmative use of these powers. The U.S. Supreme Court has never interpreted the Constitution in this way, however. Rather, the Court has viewed the Constitution as *empowering* the government to act in the name of public health, in the event a state chooses to do so (this is reminiscent of the act of licensing—for both doctors and drivers—discussed in the previous section on the "no duty to treat" principle). This, you may have guessed, is what is meant by the "negative Constitution." This doctrine holds that the Constitution does not require government to provide any goods or services whatsoever, public health or otherwise, and derives from the fact that the Constitution is phrased mainly in negative terms—for example, the Constitution's First Amendment doesn't affirmatively state that citizens have a right to free speech, it says that Congress "shall make no law" *abridging* the freedom of speech. This view of the Constitution, to paraphrase Judge Richard Posner, maintains that the drafters of the document were more concerned with what government would do *to* people rather than what government should do *for* them. In this way, the Constitution exerts a negative force that limits governmental power to restrain us as individuals, rather than compelling government to promote public health through tangible goods and services.

The application of the negative Constitution doctrine is starkly witnessed in two Supreme Court decisions—*DeShaney v. Winnebago County Department of Social Services* and *Town of Castle Rock, Colorado v. Gonzales*[26]—which both have terribly distressing facts at their core. In the *DeShaney* case, a one-year-old named Joshua DeShaney was placed in his father's custody after his parents divorced. Over the span of the next three years, multiple people—including the father's second wife and various emergency room personnel—complained to social services workers in Wisconsin that the father had been abusing Joshua physically. While county officials opened a case file and interviewed Joshua's father on multiple occasions, each time they decided that they didn't have sufficient evidence of child abuse to remove Joshua from the house and place him in court custody. When Joshua was four years old, he suffered a horrific beating at the hands of his father. He eventually survived a life-threatening coma but was left with permanent brain damage, and he was expected to live the remainder of his life in an institution for the mentally disabled. Subsequently, Joshua's father was convicted of child abuse.

Joshua's mother filed a civil rights lawsuit against the Wisconsin social services workers who failed to remove him from his abusive father's home. A 6–3 majority of the U.S. Supreme Court turned away the lawsuit in 1989, finding that under the Due Process Clause state officials had no affirmative constitutional duty to protect Joshua:

> [N]othing in the language of the Due Process Clause itself requires the State to protect the life, liberty, and property of its citizens against invasion by private actors. The Clause is phrased as a limitation on the State's power to act, not as a guarantee of certain minimal levels of safety and security. It forbids the State itself to deprive individuals of life, liberty, or property without 'due process of law,' but its language cannot fairly be extended to impose an affirmative obligation on the State to ensure that those interests do not come to harm through other means.[27]

The Court majority then went even further, ruling that while the state knew that Joshua was in danger and expressed a willingness to protect him against that danger, those facts were not enough to establish the type of affirmative duty to rescue reserved for parties who have (for purposes of the Constitution) a "special relationship."

Three Justices dissented. They argued that the State of Wisconsin, through its establishment of a child protection program, undertook a duty to intervene in Joshua's life, and that its failure to meet this duty violated the Constitution. The dissenters complained that in effect, Wisconsin's program displaced private sources of child protection but then ignored the very harm it was meant to prevent.

Sixteen years after *DeShaney*, the Supreme Court again took up the question of whether the government has a duty to affirmatively protect its citizens. Sadly, the facts in *Castle Rock v. Gonzales* are as tragic as those in *DeShaney*. Jessica Gonzales received a restraining order protecting her and her three young daughters from her husband, who was also the girls' father. One June afternoon, all three girls disappeared from in front of her home. She suspected that her husband had taken the girls in violation of the court order, a suspicion she was able to confirm through a phone call to her husband. In two initial phone conversations with the Castle Rock (Colorado) Police Department, Mrs. Gonzalez was told there was nothing the police could do and to wait until 10:00 p.m. to see if anything changed.

Nothing changed by 10:00, so Jessica again called the police, at which time she was again told to wait, this time until midnight. After this process played out yet another time, she went to her husband's apartment. Finding it empty, she went to the police station in person. Rather than attempt to locate the missing girls, the police officer who wrote up Jessica's report went to dinner. A couple hours later, Jessica's husband pulled his truck up to, and began shooting at, the Castle Rock Police Department. The police returned fire, killing him. Jessica's three daughters were found dead in the back of her husband's truck, having been murdered by their father some hours earlier.

Jessica sued the police department, claiming that its inaction violated the Constitution. Specifically, she argued that the restraining order she received was "property," and that the police effectively "took" this property in violation of the Due Process Clause's requirement that no state "deprive any person of life, liberty, or property, without due process of law." By a 7–2 margin, however, the Supreme Court ruled in favor of the town of Castle Rock, ruling that Jessica did not have an individual entitlement to enforcement of a Colorado law that requires police officers to use all reasonable means to execute restraining orders. The Court then said that even *if* it had found such an entitlement, there was uncertainty as to whether the entitlement would rise to the level of a protected "property" interest that triggers constitutional protections. According to the Court, the Due Process Clause does not protect all government "benefits," including things that government officials have discretion to grant or deny (for example, because police departments have finite resources, officers have discretion to consider whether a violation of a restraining order is too minor to justify enforcement).

Taken as a whole, the negative Constitution doctrine and the cases that apply it raise a couple important questions in the broad context of health, welfare, and safety. First, given our deep reliance on government to organize social and economic life in a way that creates conditions for us to be healthy, what do you think about a legal doctrine that holds that government has no affirmative obligation to provide services or to shield even the most vulnerable among us from another person's violence? Second, if we can't rely on the courts to check even the worst instances of government workers' failure to act, what's to prevent those same workers from "using" their inaction to harm certain people or groups (e.g., withholding important benefits from certain groups, or withholding necessary services from certain neighborhoods)?

▶ No Right to Counsel in Civil Legal Matters

The fourth and final legal doctrine discussed as a background matter concerns the ability of individuals to afford and access help when trying to enforce complex civil legal rights. This ability is, in many ways, as important as the right itself: for what good are rights to, say, food stamps and a mold-free apartment and Medicaid benefits if the holder of the rights can't actually get those things? Because the enforcement of legal rights is so important—particularly for low-income and other vulnerable populations whose reliance on social programs and services is often a quality-of-life, or life-and-death, matter—it makes sense to ask what rules and systems are in place to help people enforce their legal rights. To answer this somewhat complicated question in a succinct way, it is instructive to consider the difference between rights that attach in the area of criminal legal representation versus those that exist in the realm of civil legal assistance. It is worth noting at the outset that the U.S. is one of the only countries that completely separates access to criminal and civil legal services.

Criminal Legal Representation

Per the Sixth Amendment to the U.S. Constitution, the government is required to provide legal counsel to all federal defendants who are unable to afford their own attorneys. The right to counsel in state criminal prosecutions was established (though only for serious offences) by the U.S. Supreme Court in the well-known case of *Gideon v. Wainwright*.[28] The case started after Clarence Gideon was arrested for burglary. Indigent and unable to secure the services of private legal counsel, he asked the trial court to assign him a lawyer. Denied by the court, Gideon represented himself. He was found guilty and sentenced to five years in state prison.

Gideon appealed his conviction to the U.S. Supreme Court, claiming that the state court's refusal to grant him legal assistance violated his constitutional rights. The Supreme Court agreed to hear Gideon's case (and assigned him a highly respected lawyer). The Court eventually ruled in Gideon's favor, holding that the assistance of counsel, if desired by an indigent defendant, was a guaranteed right under the U.S. Constitution when states prosecuted people for serious crimes. Along with a new trial, Gideon received government-financed legal services, and he was cleared of all charges just a few months after the Supreme Court's landmark ruling.

Gideon v. Wainwright led to many changes in how the indigent are represented in criminal cases. For example, the decision effectively created the need for criminal lawyers employed at public expense—what are known today as public defenders—and its importance extends not only to subsequent cases concerning legal representation at trial and on appeal, but also to cases dealing with police interrogation and the well-known right to remain silent.

Civil Legal Assistance

Unlike the case for serious or high-risk criminal cases, there is no generalized right to the assistance of a lawyer in civil matters—even for the indigent and even when the most basic human needs are at stake. While states have created rights to counsel in situations dealing with the termination of parental rights, paternity, juvenile abuse, and involuntary commitment to mental health facilities, it is rare for individuals to have rights to legal assistance in very common and critical areas of civil law, including health care, immigration status, domestic violence, veterans benefits, disability needs, child custody, housing, public benefits, employment disputes, special education needs, and more. In all of these types of disputes—which can be incredibly complex and which can have life-altering consequences—individuals and families can harbor no expectation that an attorney will be on hand to help them. Instead, because they cannot afford legal fees, it is commonplace for the indigent, a growing portion of the middle class, and many small businesses to simply give up or go it alone when it comes to important civil legal needs. (Contrast this with the approach of the countries in the European Union, all of which have had a right to civil legal assistance for decades.)

Importantly, there is a legal safety net for the poorest segment of our population, who can at least try to access what are known as civil legal aid services. These services are provided by a network of publicly funded legal aid agencies, private lawyers and law firms offering free or near-free legal assistance, and law school clinics run by faculty and staffed by students. Unfortunately, however, there is far more need than there is capacity to handle that need. In the end, usually only those individuals with the lowest incomes receive assistance: some 80% of low-income individuals and 40 to 60% of middle-class individuals suffer from legal needs that go unmet. This equates to tens of millions of people who cannot access the legal assistance they need to save their homes, their jobs, their rightful public benefits, and the like.[29]

As a matter of pure funding, the U.S. Congress is most to blame for the enormous gap that exists between civil legal needs and resources. Congress holds the purse strings of the Legal Services Corporation (LSC), a not-for-profit corporation established by federal law in 1974 as the single largest funder of civil legal aid for low-income Americans. In today's dollars, LSC's congressional appropriation in 1976 was about $479,000,000; in 2015, that number was $375,000,000. But this $100,000,000 reduction does not even tell the whole story, for over the 40-year-period just referred to, need has soared—meaning that LSC's budget should be much higher than even its inflation-adjusted 1976 budget just to keep pace with increased need over time.

The link between civil legal problems and health is underlined by the Community Needs and Services Study, an examination of the civil justice experiences of the American public.[30] According to the study, two-thirds of adults in a middle-sized American city experienced at least 1 of 12 different categories of civil justice situations in the previous 18 months. Notably, the average number of situations reported rested at 3.3, and poor people, blacks, and Hispanics were more likely to report civil justice situations than were middle- or high-income earners and whites. The most commonly reported situations concerned employment issues, government benefits, health insurance, and housing. The study uncovered significant connections between civil justice situations and health: respondents indicated that nearly half of the situations resulted in feelings of fear, a loss of confidence, damage to physical or mental health, or verbal or physical violence or threats of violence. In fact, adverse impacts on health were the most common negative consequence, reported for 27% of situations. Also important is the fact many of those who responded indicated that they didn't even know that the problems they were experiencing were rightly considered "legal" in nature. The link between civil legal needs and health will be more fully explored in the chapter on existing safety net programs and legal protections.

▶ Conclusion

As evidenced by the legal doctrines described in this chapter, the nation's health has much more than just social support deficiencies and luck working against it; it has long-standing, deeply rooted legal doctrines to account for, as well. Creating universal health insurance coverage? That could easily be done by way of a federal statute, assuming the political will was present. A shift in national spending priorities away from downstream medical procedures in favor of more upstream social care? In other nations similar to our own, this is the norm, so it can't be that difficult. And universal health insurance and social determinants of health are, at least, relatively common discussion topics among policymakers. But realigning bedrock legal principles that in some cases don't even conjure up the notion of "health consequences" for most people? That is a true challenge. One of the aims of this text is simply to help lay people to understand that things like "suspect classifications" and the "negative Constitution" are important legal principles that pertain to the nation's health. After you've read the text in its entirety, it is our hope that it will become one of your aims, as well.

References

1. Hurley v. Eddingfield, 59 N.E. 1058 (Ind. 1901).
2. Reinhardt U. The debate that wasn't: the public and the Clinton health care plan. In: Aaron H., ed. *The Problem That Won't Go Away: Reforming U.S. Health Care Financing.* Washington, DC: Brookings Institution; 1996:70–109, 102.

3. Mendes E. More than three in 10 in U.S. put off treatment due to cost. *Gallup News.* December 12, 2014. Available at: http://news.gallup.com/poll/159218/three-put-off-treatment-due-cost .aspx?utm_source=alert&utm_medium=email&utm_campaign=syndication&utm _content=morelink&utm_term=USA%20-%20Wellbeing%20-%20Well-Being%20Index.

4. Nice JA. No scrutiny whatsoever: deconstitutionalization of poverty law, dual rules of law and dialogic default. *Fordham Urban Law Journal.* 2008;35:630–631.

5. *See* Craig v. Boren, 429 U.S. 190 (1976).

6. United States v. Carolene Products Co., 304 U.S. 144, 152–153 n. 4 (1938).

7. Korematsu v. United States, 323 U.S. 214, 216 (1944).

8. Craig v. Boren, 429 U.S. 190, 197 (1976).

9. For a summary of the Court's analyses in determining suspect and quasi-suspect classes, *see* Rose H. The poor as a suspect class under the Equal Protection Clause: an open constitutional question. *Nova Law Review.* 2010;48:419–420.

10. Massachusetts Board of Retirement v. Murgia, 427 U.S. 307 (US SC 1976).

11. Romer v. Evans, 517 U.S. 620, 635 (1996).

12. Roe v. Wade, 410 U.S. 113, 152–153 (1973).

13. Davis MF. *Brutal Need: Lawyers and the Welfare Rights Movement, 1960–1973.* New Haven, CT: Yale University Press; 1993: Chapters 1–2.

14. King v. Smith, 392 U.S. 309, 332–333 (1968).

15. Shapiro v. Thompson, 394 U.S. 618, 633 (1969).

16. Davis MF. *Brutal Need: Lawyers and the Welfare Rights Movement, 1960–1973.* New Haven, CT: Yale University Press; 1993:80.

17. Goldberg v. Kelly, 397 U.S. 254, 262 (1970).

18. Goldberg v. Kelly, 397 U.S. 254, 262 (1970).

19. Dandridge v. Williams, 397 U.S. 471, 486–487 (1970).

20. San Antonio Independent School Dist. v. Rodriguez, 411 U.S. 1, 29 (1973). The Court also held that education is not a fundamental right, but went on to say that the children were receiving an education, even if it was substandard.

21. Davis MF. *Brutal Need: Lawyers and the Welfare Rights Movement, 1960–1973.* New Haven, CT: Yale University Press; 1993: Chapter 9.

22. *See* Nice JA. No scrutiny whatsoever: deconstitutionalization of poverty law, dual rules of law and dialogic default. *Fordham Urban Law Journal.* 2008;35:633.

23. Rose H. The poor as a suspect class under the Equal Protection Clause: an open constitutional question. *Nova Law Review.* 210;34(2):408.

24. Nice JA. No scrutiny whatsoever: deconstitutionalization of poverty law, dual rules of law and dialogic default. *Fordham Urban Law Journal.* 2008;35:648.

25. Romer v. Evans, 517 U.S. 620, 635 (1996). *See* Dyson MR. Rethinking *Rodriguez* after *Citizens United*: the poor as a suspect class in high-poverty schools. *Georgetown Journal on Poverty Law & Policy.* 2016;24(1),1-58.

26. 489 U.S. 189 (1989) and 545 U.S. 748 (2005), respectively.

27. 489 U.S. at 195.

28. 372 U.S. 335 (1963).

29. Legal Services Corporation. *The Justice Gap: Measuring the Unmet Civil Legal Needs of Low-Income Americans.* Prepared by NORC at the University of Chicago for Legal Services Corporation. Washington, DC; 2017. Available at: https://www.lsc.gov/sites/default/files /images/TheJusticeGap-FullReport.pdf.

30. Rebecca L. Sandefur. Accessing justice in the contemporary USA: findings from the Community Needs and Services Study. Chicago, IL: American Bar Foundation; 2014. Available at: http:// www.americanbarfoundation.org/uploads/cms/documents/sandefur_accessing_justice_in _the_contemporary_usa._aug._2014.pdf.

CHAPTER 2

The Effects of Discrimination and Implicit Bias on Health and Health Care

LEARNING OBJECTIVES

By the end of this chapter you will be able to:

- Describe the lasting effects of historical discrimination and segregation on health and health care.
- Explain the meaning and health-harming effects of implicit bias.

▶ Introduction

In the chapter on social and structural barriers to health, we describe in detail many social factors that directly or indirectly contribute to poor health, or at least make it exceedingly difficult for vulnerable individuals and communities to achieve optimal health. In this chapter we single out two such factors—discrimination and bias—for separate treatment. Unfortunately, the nation's discriminatory history has left an indelible mark on the health of populations of color, and thus it serves as an important backdrop to subsequent discussions about social systems that lead to health disparities and injustices.

We note at the outset that blacks are hardly the only group that has suffered health-harming discrimination and marginalization. Other racial groups, ethnic minorities, the impoverished, religious minorities, people with disabilities, women, and others have all been excluded from the healthful benefits associated with full participation in society, and we discuss many of these groups in the next chapter in the context of health disparities. That said, we mainly focus in this chapter on blacks, due to the relatively intense harms that discrimination and bias have caused in this population.

Race-based discrimination can be expressed on three different levels: interpersonal, internalized, and structural/institutional. Interpersonal racism is unfair treatment of a person or group by individuals (e.g., denying a person a job or an apartment rental based on the person's race); internalized racism occurs when victims of racism internalize prejudicial attitudes toward themselves and/or their racial or ethnic group, resulting in, among other things, stress and a loss of self-esteem; and structural racism refers to prejudices that are built into policies, laws, and societal practices.[1] Structural racism can be particularly wicked: it can be rooted in overt racism from decades or centuries past, but can result in even unintentional discrimination today as policies and practices are passed on through the generations.

In addition, not all racism is conscious. "Implicit bias" refers to "bias in judgment and/or behavior that results from subtle cognitive processes (e.g., implicit attitudes and implicit stereotypes) that often operate at a level below conscious awareness and without intentional control."[2] In other words:

> it is the automatic association of stereotypes with particular groups. These automatic associations become problematic when they are assumed to predict real world behavior and when decision making is based on them. Automatic negative associations with stereotypes or implicit racial attitudes, while existing in the unconscious, become displayed through the individual's behavior. These behaviors are often apparent in microaggressions, which are 'brief and commonplace daily verbal, behavioral, and environmental indignities, whether intentional or unintentional, that communicate hostile, derogatory, or negative racial slights and insults to the target person or group.'[3]

As described below, evidence suggests that unconscious biases are deeply rooted and remain widespread.[4]

Regardless of whether race-based discrimination is interpersonal, internalized, structural, intentional, or subconscious, it can raise the risk of a host of health conditions, both emotional and physical.[5] Furthermore, at the same time that discrimination has been woven into the fabric of society, it can be further sustained by weakening the legal machinery that enforces civil rights laws. For example, a review of the first proposed federal budget put forth by the Trump Administration reveals that it is aiming to broadly reduce the promotion and protection of civil rights. The budget proposes to disband the Labor Department's Office of Federal Contract Compliance Programs, which has some 600 employees and fights discrimination among federal contractors; it would gut the Environmental Protection Agency's environmental justice program, which combats pollution-related threats in minority communities; it would significantly cut staffing in the Education Department's Office of Civil Rights; and it would shift the manpower in the Justice Department that aims to curb civil rights abuses in police departments across the country.[6] These types of policy shifts can result in both direct and indirect risks to health. At the time of this writing, it is not clear how many of these proposals will be implemented.

This chapter is devised of two parts. We first describe in broad strokes the legacy of historical health care discrimination. We then describe more fully the concept of implicit bias and discuss its implications for health.

▶ The Legacy of Historical Discrimination In Health Care

There is simply no doing justice to the topic of health care discrimination in a handful of pages; the description and legacy of overt, legally sanctioned discrimination and segregation in health care are simply too massive to document in a short primer on health justice. Indeed, the most authoritative treatise on the subject—Michael Byrd and Linda Clayton's *An American Health Dilemma*[7]—is two volumes and nearly 1,500 pages. There are additional books and many, many scholarly articles on the subject, as well. Thus, what we can provide here is, relatively speaking, a thumbnail overview and summary.

The roots of interpersonal and structural racism in the United States are buried in the earliest experiences of Native Americans and African Americans. Both groups suffered genocide, enslavement, and legalized racial oppression at the hands of those who colonized North America. This treatment in and of itself, however—as horrible as it was—is not what locked in subsequent centuries of race-based discrimination and segregation. Rather, this oppression set in motion in the U.S. an evolving and durable belief system that perpetuated the myth that people of color—black people, in particular—were inferior to white people.[8] This had the long-term effects of legitimizing slavery and relegating blacks to a lower social, financial, and educational status relative to whites. This belief system has been resistant enough to survive the Civil War, passage and implementation of the Constitution's Thirteenth and Fourteenth Amendments, the Civil Rights Movement in the 1960s, and the election of the first black president.

The interpersonal and structural racism that permeated all facets of American life before and after the Civil War were, unsurprisingly, no less pronounced in the health care system. Just as there were separate schoolrooms for blacks and whites, there were health care facilities on plantations that only slave laborers were forced to use. Just as there were separate transportation systems, there were separate hospitals (hospitals run by the U.S. Department of Veterans Affairs, for example, were not desegregated until 1954). Just as there were separate bathrooms, there were separate medical, nursing, and dental schools—once blacks were permitted to attend these schools, of course; as of the mid-1930s, only two medical schools would admit blacks. Just as there were separate drinking fountains, there were separate physician practices. Just as there were racially segregated neighborhoods, there were separate professional medical societies (black people were effectively excluded from the American Medical Association right up until the Civil Rights Era).

Although these separate health systems existed through the better part of the twentieth century, the white majority's interest in the health of blacks underwent something of a shift around 1900. Recognizing that white health was affected by the health of the broader population—germs did not segregate on the basis of a host's race, after all—medical professionals decided that minority health was also important. However, this "care" was decidedly paternalistic. For example, forced sterilization of black women was not uncommon after the American Civil War (when whites worried about a growing black population that sought enhanced legal rights and protections). The practice of forced sterilization continued until the 1960s.

In terms of undisguised health care racism, however, little compares with the Tuskegee syphilis experiment. Undertaken by the U.S. Public Health Service and the private Tuskegee Institute, the 40-year study aimed to understand the effects of untreated syphilis on black men in Alabama. Study subjects went untreated because researchers never informed them of the actual purpose of the study; rather, the men were told that they were being treated for "bad blood." As a result, the men were never given the chance to provide informed consent. The nontreatment continued even after penicillin became the drug of choice for syphilis in 1947 since, if the men being studied were actually cared for, researchers could no longer study the bodily effects of untreated syphilis. While the federal government eventually apologized for conducting the study and paid an out-of-court settlement to participants and their families, the Tuskegee study's legacy continues to resonate today. Minority distrust of government-sponsored health services and of participation in human subject research is relatively high, which limits minorities' willingness to participate in important therapeutic trials. In fact, a 1997 study of multiple black focus groups concerning their views on medical research and the Tuskegee study found that, among other things, distrust of medical researchers posed a substantial barrier to study recruitment.

Another notable event—notable because nothing else like it exists in twentieth century statutory law—was passage in 1946 of the federal Hospital Survey and Construction Act, also referred to as the Hill-Burton Act after the two senators who sponsored the legislation. The Hill-Burton Act authorized the use of federal funds for states to build new hospitals (and refurbish old ones) in the aftermath of World War II, provided that hospitals cared for a "reasonable volume" of patients who were unable to pay for services. As a matter of financing, Hill-Burton was a powerhouse: in the 30 years after passage, the law subsidized the construction of 40% of hospital beds across the country. However, Hill-Burton—passed only eight years before *Brown vs. Board of Education* was decided—is perhaps best known for a provision that explicitly permitted federal financing of discriminatory practices:

> a hospital will be made available to all persons residing in [its] territorial area . . ., without discrimination on account of race, creed, or color, but an exception shall be made in cases where separate hospital facilities are provided for separate population groups, if the plan makes equitable provision on the basis of need for facilities and services of like quality for each such group.[9]

This racist federal law survived for 17 years before it was ruled unconstitutional in the case of *Simkins v. Moses H. Cone Memorial Hospital*,[10] which has been referred to as the "Brown v. Board of Education" of health care.[11]

Congress has never passed a comprehensive civil rights statute for health care comparable to, say, Title VII of the Civil Rights Act of 1964 (prohibiting employers from discriminating against employees on the basis of race and color, among other things), the Voting Rights Act of 1965, the Fair Housing Act (passed as Title VIII of the Civil Rights Act of 1968), and similar landmark laws whose intentions are to make certain aspects of society more equal. Combating discrimination in health care did get a boost in the 1960s, however, by way of Title VI of the 1964 Civil Rights Act. Title VI prohibits discrimination on the basis of race, color, or national origin by programs and activities that receive federal financial assistance.[12] The statute passed by Congress outlaws intentional discrimination, while the regulations implementing the statute go further, reaching conduct and practices that, even if unintentional, nonetheless have a discriminatory impact on members of minority groups. While Title VI remains deeply important to efforts to stamp out race-based discrimination in health care,[13] the ability of individuals to enforce their rights under the law was deeply undercut by a controversial U.S. Supreme Court decision in 2001.[14] (In the case of *Alexander v. Sandoval*, the Court ruled that the discriminatory impact regulation mentioned above may not be enforced by the very individuals suffering the discrimination; rather, according to the Court, only the federal government has enforcement authority.) In addition to Title VI, the Medicare and Medicaid programs are important pieces in the health justice puzzle, providing health insurance coverage to some of the nation's most vulnerable populations; the federal Emergency Medical Treatment and Active Labor Act effectively requires that everyone—regardless of race, health insurance status, or ability to pay—presenting at a hospital emergency room be screened and treated for an emergency medical condition; and the Affordable Care Act has made important strides in moving the nation closer to universal health insurance coverage.

Needless to say, it is of paramount importance that the health system is no longer actively segregated and that there are federal laws that aim to root out health care discrimination, reduce health and health care disparities, and promote health justice. Yet it is equally important to understand that racial discrimination in health care persists, that the health care system operates in a broader context of societal structural racism, and that institutional racism in one sector can reinforce it in others.[15] Perhaps most important in the latter regard is racial residential segregation—i.e., the physical separation of groups into different geographic areas based on race, which can easily shape individual and familial living experiences as far down as the neighborhood level. (Residential segregation—among all the various forms of structural racism—is so profound in the context of health equity because it can easily lead to educational and occupational segregation, as well. Thus, marginalized groups are subjected not only to lower-quality neighborhoods, but to lower-quality schools and jobs, as well. As you will learn in the chapter on social and structural barriers to health, education and job quality are key predictors of overall health.)

Historically, race-based living patterns were shaped by two practices. First, the use of "restrictive covenants"—a clause in a property deed or lease that limits what the owner can do with the property—effectively prohibited blacks from owning, leasing, or living in certain homes or entire neighborhoods. These covenants were used with regularity until the U.S. Supreme Court ruled them unconstitutional in 1948.[16] Second, the Federal Housing Administration, an agency that, among other things, insures mortgages, began "redlining" in the mid-1930s. The term derives from the agency's proclivity to mark maps with red lines to depict neighborhoods where mortgages should be denied to people of color, thus ensuring many all-white neighborhoods. Redlining was eventually prohibited in 1968.[17] Although restrictive covenants and redlining have been outlawed, racial residential segregation is hardly a thing of the past: recent census data indicate that the average white person in metropolitan America lives in a neighborhood that is 75% white, while a typical black person lives in a neighborhood that is 35% white and as much as 45% black.[18]

If—as alluded to in the Introduction to this book and discussed further in the chapter on social and structural barriers to health—health is more a function of one's zip code than genetic code, then racial residential segregation matters enormously for purposes of health justice. Indeed:

> the literature on racial residential segregation and poor health examines several direct and indirect pathways through which structural racism harms health, including the high concentration of dilapidated housing in neighborhoods that people of color reside in, the substandard quality of the social and built environment, exposure to pollutants and toxins, limited opportunities for high-quality education and decent employment, and restricted access to quality health care. Health outcomes associated with residential segregation documented among black Americans include adverse birth outcomes, increased exposure to air pollutants, decreased longevity, increased risk of chronic disease, and increased rates of homicide and other crime. Residential segregation is thus a foundation of structural racism and contributes to racialized health inequities.[19]

In case these claims are too broad to really resonate, consider a 2017 study in the *Internal Medicine Journal of the American Medical Association*. The study points to evidence that blacks living in racially segregated neighborhoods experience higher blood pressure than people living in relatively diverse areas.[20] Furthermore, the act of moving from segregated communities to integrated ones was associated with a decrease in blood pressure. Consider also a study that reviewed admission patterns for heart attack patients at some 2,400 U.S. hospitals. The study considered the relationship between skin color and admission to "high-mortality hospitals," defined as those hospitals with the top-third highest mortality rates. The researchers found that black patients were more likely to be admitted to high-mortality hospitals even when they lived closer to low-mortality hospitals. This finding indicates that blacks continue to be directed to lower-quality facilities contrary to medical protocol, which generally dictates that people suffering heart attacks be directed to the closest hospital.[21] These are just two specific examples, among many. Why are there so many examples linking racialized housing patterns and health outcomes? A well-known 1980 study of the 171 largest cities in the U.S. sums it up rather succinctly: the *worst* urban context in which whites typically reside is considerably better than the *average* environments of black communities.[22]

Racial residential segregation is not the only type of structural racism that works across sectors to harm health. The Flint, Michigan, water crisis, in which the majority-black city was subjected to lead-contaminated drinking water by apathetic city and state health officials, is an example of environmental racism; targeted sales of cigarettes, alcohol, and high-fructose beverages to low-income communities of color is a form of structural racism; and state laws that purport to root out "voter fraud" at the expense of minority voting rights is a type of structural discrimination.[23] These and other structural pathways must be included when discussing health-harming discrimination, and we explore them more fully in the chapter on social and structural barriers to health.

Taking together everything you've read thus far, it should come as no surprise that blacks live sicker and die sooner than whites. In fact, every 7 minutes in the U.S. a black person dies prematurely from poor health.[24] Discrimination and the chronic stress that often results from it play a substantial role in this morbidity and mortality. (To see a series of resources measuring and depicting everyday discrimination, search for Professor David Williams' "Measuring Discrimination Resource.") While researchers are just beginning to understand the full range of physical, mental, and emotional responses that occur in response to ritualized structural and interpersonal race discrimination, what is apparent is that persistent stress can lead to increased rates of hypertension, diabetes, cancer, stroke, kidney disease, maternal death, and more. The next chapter, which covers health disparities, picks up on this thread and describes the ways in which certain population groups suffer disproportionately from poor health. For the time being, we leave the topic of overt discrimination to focus on its pernicious relative—implicit bias.

▶ Implicit Bias and Its Connection to Health

Recall from the beginning of this chapter the discussion about the earliest instances of racial oppression against Native Americans and blacks, and how that oppression laid the groundwork for a cascading, multigenerational belief system premised on the idea of white superiority. While this type of overt racism is no longer the norm, it does have a distant relative that has been informed by history and infects everyone: implicit bias. "Bias" refers to an inclination toward a person or group compared with another person or group, and in this instance, "implicit" means that the inclination operates at a level below conscious awareness. Research shows that these "automatic beliefs" are deeply held and can guide behaviors in ways that contribute to persistent inequality,[25] and a federal court was blunt in its assessment that implicit bias is "no less corrosive of the achievement of equality" than explicit and overt discrimination.[26] What makes implicit biases so enduring is that generally speaking, individuals consciously hold nonprejudiced beliefs and do not realize that they are being motivated by implicit biases.

You can probably think of many ways that implicit biases could negatively influence health. To get you started, consider a few possibilities. Might clinicians act on the basis of implicit biases when recommending treatment options? (And would it even be reasonable to expect health care providers' biases *not* to seep into the snap decisions they often have to make in high-pressure environments such as hospital emergency departments?[27]) Could officials charged with administering health programs make policy decisions based on unconscious views? Isn't it likely that instructors and mentors in the health professions will pass along their biases to the next generation of care providers, thereby perpetuating unequal treatment? Before discussing more fully the pathways between implicit biases and health, we pause to briefly describe how implicit bias is measured.

Measuring Implicit Bias

The Implicit Association Test (IAT), developed in 1998, is the most widely-used measure of implicit bias. The IAT is a computerized test that records the time it takes for a participant to associate two categories of people (e.g., Black/White, Gay/Straight, Male/Female) with positive or negative adjectives (e.g., "wonderful," "horrible," "cooperative," "difficult"). The IAT is based on the theory that a quick association time reveals the participant's true feelings about the two categories of people, as it takes longer to respond if they are actually working to override their automatic association.[28] The racial attitudes IAT is available online and has been taken millions of times. Cumulative results of these tests reveal that white participants have a pro-white bias, to varying degrees.[29] Although the IAT has been criticized for being unreliable—participants frequently get different results in subsequent re-takings—it remains the foundation for much of the research around implicit bias.

One bias measurement tool popular in bioethics is called the "assumption method"[30] (it is given this name because there is an assumption from the outset that individuals being measured are explicitly motivated to disregard factors such as race). The assumption method adapts what's known in health care as the "clinical vignette"—a common teaching tool in health education that tests a student's knowledge of symptoms, diagnosis, and treatment options using a hypothetical patient fact pattern. In the assumption method, the only difference between two clinical vignettes is the characteristic that is the subject of the bias, such as the race of the patient. Differences in diagnoses or treatment between otherwise identical vignettes are attributed to bias.[31]

How Implicit Bias Affects the Provider-Patient Relationship

In one of the first studies of implicit bias in health care, a majority of physicians agreed that their own implicit race bias may affect their treatment decisions.[32] This intuition is largely borne out by the evidence, as most studies find that health care providers possess some level of bias against black people, and that bias, rooted in stereotype, often animates diagnosis decisions or treatment recommendations.[33] Implicit bias can go so far as to cause providers to ignore the facts in front of them, such as in the following example:

> At a well-known academic medical center, a child presented with difficulty breathing that baffled the care team. The team of physicians were [sic] agonizing over a light box, reviewing the patient's X-rays, puzzled because they couldn't determine a diagnosis. Another physician just passing through looked at the X-rays and immediately said, "cystic fibrosis." The team was tripped up by the patient's race, which was black, and that the patient had a "white disease."[34]

On the subject of treatment recommendations, a study found that pediatricians' biases lead them to prescribe less pain medication to black children than white children. Another study demonstrated that physicians are less inclined to recommend blood-clot surgery for black patients based on the "perception" that they are not as cooperative about treatment recommendations as are white patients.[35] At the same time, another study of pediatricians treating Native American children found that, despite IAT results showing physician bias against Native Americans, there was little difference in treatment recommendations for asthma and pain control based on race.[36]

Implicit bias can also negatively affect the quality of the relationship between provider and patient, with race-biased providers receiving lower marks in communication and interpersonal treatment from black patients than white ones.[37] Patients who perceive that their providers are biased against them, even if that bias is not overt, may not trust their provider and thus may be less likely to adhere to treatment regimes.[38]

Whether physicians' implicit biases result in adverse health outcomes for their patients is less clear. While a 2014 blood pressure study found implicit bias among health care providers, it also found that it had no impact on health outcomes for black and Latino patients.[39] But in a study of patients with a disabling spinal cord injury, pro-white, anti-black bias among physicians was associated—among black patients—with greater depression, lower levels of life satisfaction, and more difficulty integrating socially.[40]

How Implicit Bias Can Shape Systems and Policy

When, for example, health care providers act upon their biases, it can affect their relationship with patients, influence treatment decisions, and ultimately contribute to health disparities. But when unconscious attitudes shape systems and policy, the effect is, naturally, felt on a much larger scale, and the results can undermine health equity. For example, implicit bias may explain why the amount of cash assistance available to low-income people depends more on the state in which a family lives, rather than the family's experience of poverty. (As you will read in the chapter on social and structural barriers to health, governmental cash assistance is a critical lifeline to health for many low-income individuals and families.) The Urban Institute—an economic and social policy research organization in Washington, DC—found that, under the Temporary Assistance to Needy Families (TANF) program, states with larger populations of white people provide more cash assistance, and have more generous access rules, than states that have larger black populations. Thus, low-income black families are more likely to live in states with more restrictive policies for obtaining or keeping TANF benefits.[41]

Systems and policies designed to spark the use of health information technology can also introduce bias into provider-patient relationships. In one electronic medical record system, an airplane icon is displayed for so-called "frequent flyers": patients with chronic physical, mental, or substance use conditions who frequently use emergency departments or psychiatric crisis centers. Usually used pejoratively in a health care context, "frequent flyers" are assumed to be problem patients. (A better term for patients who require relatively high levels of health care is "high need, high cost.") Rather than provide care based on the patient's medical problems, a health care provider using this particular electronic medical record system may instead react to the icon—perhaps without ever having even spoken to the patient— and make assumptions based upon the "frequent flyer" designation. If providers begin encounters with patients with a "problem patient" stereotype in their mind, they may fail to diagnose genuine medical issues or fail to provide quality care.[42]

Similarly, medical education may unwittingly reinforce or encourage implicit bias, thus indoctrinating new generations of health care providers into unconscious stereotyping. For example, clinical vignettes that rely upon racial or gender stereotypes may encourage students to draw conclusions based on these stereotypes rather than on the individual characteristics of patients.[43] Negative role modeling may also contribute to systemic bias in health care. During their formative training years, medical students witness physicians acting upon their implicit biases and may replicate this "hidden curriculum" in practice. For example, physicians may assume that patients with limited English proficiency are more difficult to treat because of the time required to engage an interpreter, and thus may provide less information to those patients in an effort to save time. Medical students, told in class to provide high-quality care to all patients, receive a different message when they see physicians cut corners as a result of their biases.[44]

Efforts to Combat Implicit Bias in Health Care

Implicit bias can negatively affect individual health and ultimately increase health disparities across groups. Yet because it operates on an unconscious level and is often contrary to consciously held beliefs, what can be done to combat it? Rather than pretend that implicit bias does not exist—and, in fact, we all harbor these types of biases—experts encourage people to equate implicit bias with a bad habit that must be acknowledged, analyzed, and then overcome by a nonprejudiced response. Methods include consciously replacing stereotypes with counter-examples, or using role-playing games in which individuals imagine themselves in the position of the victim of bias.[45]

As it turns out, implicit bias among health care providers has been reduced when providers are given more opportunities for meeting individual members of different groups in a positive, unpressured setting.[46] Individuation—where medical students are taught to consider a patient as an individual rather than as a member of a group—prioritizes the patient's individual characteristics over their membership. Making individuation a routine part of medical education and care delivery could decrease bias in high-pressure settings, like crowded emergency rooms, where providers must react quickly.[47] And innovations such as "implicit bias rounds," in which health care providers consider how implicit bias may have detrimentally affected their past care of a patient, can help providers understand the role of bias in their practice.[48]

Although it may seem obvious, health care providers must be encouraged to follow clinical guidelines for care rather than making assumptions about, for example, whether a patient will adhere to a treatment regime based on prevalent stereotypes about a group's level of cooperation.[49] Because implicit bias has been shown to influence the interpersonal relationship between health care providers and patients, the reduction of behavior based on bias may serve as one step towards reducing health disparities and increasing health equity.

▶ Conclusion

This chapter scratches the surface of two of the more unsavory social determinants of health: discrimination and bias against people based on an immutable trait or membership in a particular group. These health-related social factors, as you will see in the next two chapters, braid together with many others to result in a raft of various health disparities. (Make no mistake, these disparities are not limited to health care delivery or to race: as noted previously, research also points to disparities in health care access, diagnosis, and outcomes based on socioeconomic status, physical and mental disability, gender, sexual orientation, geographic location, and more.) But we singled out discrimination and bias to provide backdrop and context and to call them out for what they are: an enduring component of a society and health system that relegate far too many fellow human beings to the fringes of well-being. There is little question that as a whole, society is making progress: the causes of health disparities and health inequities are relatively new topics of study, and there is an effort afoot to mainstream the idea that implicit biases are both widespread and remediable. But more can, and should, be done to combat discrimination and prejudice.

References

1. Braveman P, Arkin E, Orleans T, Proctor D, Plough A. *What Is Health Equity? And What Difference Does a Definition Make?* Brooklyn, NY: Robert Wood Johnson Foundation; 2017. Available at: https://www.rwjf.org/en/library/research/2017/05/what-is-health-equity-.html.
2. Casey PM, Warren RK, Cheesman FL, Elek JK. *Helping Courts Address Implicit Bias: Resources for Education B-2.* National Center for State Courts; 2012. Available at: http://www.ncsc.org/~/media/Files/PDF/Topics/Gender%20and%20Racial%20Fairness/IB_report_033012.ashx.
3. Benfer EA. Health justice: a framework (and call to action) for the elimination of health inequity and social justice. *American University Law Review.* 2015;65(2):278–279 (internal footnotes omitted).
4. Braveman P, Arkin E, Orleans T, Proctor D, Plough A. *What Is Health Equity? And What Difference Does a Definition Make?* Brooklyn, NY: Robert Wood Johnson Foundation; 2017. Available at: https://www.rwjf.org/en/library/research/2017/05/what-is-health-equity-.html.
5. Benfer EA. Health justice: a framework (and call to action) for the elimination of health inequity and social justice. *American University Law Review.* 2015;65(2):275, 283; Silverstein J. How racism is bad for our bodies. *The Atlantic.* March 12, 2013. Available at: http://www.theatlantic.com/health/archive/2013/03/how-racism-is-bad-forour-bodies/273911.
6. Eilperin J, Brown E, Fears D. Trump administration plans to minimize civil rights efforts in agencies. *The Washington Post.* May 29, 2017. Available at: https://www.washingtonpost.com/politics/trump-administration-plans-to-minimize-civil-rights-efforts-in-agencies/2017/05/29/922fc1b2-39a7-11e7-a058-ddbb23c75d82_story.html?hpid=hp_rhp-top-table-main_civilrights-737pm%3Ahomepage%2Fstory&utm_term=.b9f275e47887.
7. Byrd WM, Clayton LA. *An American Health Dilemma: A Medical History of African Americans and the Problem of Race.* New York, NY: Routledge; 2000.
8. Equal Justice Initiative. *Slavery in America: The Montgomery Slave Trade.* Available at: https://eji.org/reports/slavery-in-america.
9. 42 U.S.C. § 291e(f) (1946).
10. Simkins v. Moses H. Cone Memorial Hospital, 323 F.2d 959 (4th Cir.1963), cert. den. 376 U.S. 938 (1964).
11. Smith DB. *Health Care Divided: Race and Healing a Nation.* Ann Arbor, MI: The University of Michigan Press; 1999.
12. 42 U.S.C. § 2000d (1964).
13. Rosenbaum S, Schmucker S. Viewing health equity through a legal lens: Title VI of the 1964 Civil Rights Act. *Journal of Health Policy, Politics, and Law.* June 2017;42(5):771.
14. Rosenbaum S, Teitelbaum J. Civil rights enforcement in the modern healthcare system: reinvigorating the role of the federal government in the aftermath of *Alexander v. Sandoval. Yale Journal of Health Policy, Law, and Ethics.* 2003;3(2): article 1.
15. Bailey ZD, Krieger N, Agénor M, Graves J, Linos N, Bassett MT. Structural racism and health inequities in the U.S.A.: evidence and interventions. *Lancet.* 2017;389:1453–1463.
16. Shelley v. Kraemer, 334 U.S. 1 (1948).
17. Title VIII of the Civil Rights Act of 1968, Pub. L. 90-284, 82 Stat. 73 (1968).
18. Bailey ZD, Krieger N, Agénor M, Graves J, Linos N, Bassett MT. Structural racism and health inequities in the U.S.A.: evidence and interventions. *Lancet.* 2017;389:1455–1456.
19. Bailey ZD, Krieger N, Agénor M, Graves J, Linos N, Bassett MT. Structural racism and health inequities in the U.S.A.: evidence and interventions. *Lancet.* 2017;389:1456–1457.

20. Kershaw KN, Robinson WR, Gorden-Larsen P. Association of changes in neighborhood-level racial residential segregation with changes in blood pressure among black adults. *JAMA Internal Medicine.* 2017;177(7):996–1002. Available at: https://jamanetwork.com/journals/jamainternalmedicine/article-abstract/2626858.

21. Sarrazin MV, Campbell M, Rosenthal, GE. Racial differences in hospital use after acute myocardial infarction: does residential segregation play a role? *Health Affairs.* March/April 2009;28(2):w368–78.

22. Sampson RJ, Wilson WJ. Toward a theory of race, crime, and urban inequality. In: Hagan J, Peterson RD, eds. *Crime and Inequality.* Stanford, CA: Stanford University Press; 1995: 37–56.

23. Bailey ZD, Krieger N, Agénor M, Graves J, Linos N, Bassett MT. Structural racism and health inequities in the U.S.A.: evidence and interventions. *Lancet.* 2017;389:1453–1463.

24. Williams DR. Social sources of racial disparities in health. *Health Affairs.* 2005;24(2):325–334.

25. Devine PG, Forscher PS, Austin AJ, Cox WTL. Long-term reduction in implicit race bias: a prejudice habit-breaking intervention. *Journal of Experimental Social Psychology.* 2012;48(6): 1267–1278.

26. Woods v. City of Greensboro, 2017 WL 174898 (4th Cir. May 5, 2017) (finding the lower court erred in dismissing minority-owned business's claim of discrimination based on implicit bias).

27. Johnson TJ, Hickey RW, Switzer GE, et al. The impact of cognitive stressors in the emergency department on physician implicit bias. *Academic Emergency Medicine.* 2016;23(3):297–305.

28. Matthew DB. *Just Medicine: A Cure for Racial Inequality in American Health Care.* New York, NY: New York University Press; 2016.

29. Project Implicit. Available at: https://implicit.harvard.edu/implicit/. *See also* Mooney C. Across America, whites are biased and they don't even know it. *The Washington Post.* December 8, 2014. Available at: https://www.washingtonpost.com/news/wonk/wp/2014/12/08/across-america-whites-are-biased-and-they-dont-even-know-it/?utm_term=.3af98c51a7cc.

30. FitzGerald C, Hurst S. Implicit bias in healthcare professionals: a systematic review. *BMC Medical Ethics.* 2017;18(19):1–18.

31. FitzGerald C, Hurst S. Implicit bias in healthcare professionals: a systematic review. *BMC Medical Ethics.* 2017;18(19):1–18.

32. Green AR, Carney DR, Pallin DJ, et al. Implicit bias among physicians and its prediction of thrombolysis decisions for black and white patients. *Journal of General Internal Medicine.* 2007;22(9):1231–1238.

33. Hall WJ. Implicit racial/ethnic bias among health care professionals and its influence on health care outcomes: a systematic review. *American Journal of Public Health.* 2015;105(12): e60–e76.

34. The Joint Commission. Implicit bias in health care. *Quick Safety.* April 2016;23. Available at: https://www.jointcommission.org/assets/1/23/Quick_Safety_Issue_23_Apr_2016.pdf.

35. Sabin JA. The influence of implicit bias on treatment recommendations for 4 common pediatric conditions: pain, urinary tract infection, attention deficit hyperactivity disorder, and asthma. *American Journal of Public Health.* 2012;102(5):988–995; Green AR, Carney DR, Pallin DJ, et al. Implicit bias among physicians and its prediction of thrombolysis decisions for black and white patients. *Journal of General Internal Medicine.* 2007;22(9):1231–1238.

36. Puumala SE. The role of bias by emergency department providers in care for American Indian children. *Medical Care.* 2016;54(6):562–569.

37. Blair IV. An investigation of associations between clinicians' ethnic or racial bias and hypertension treatment, medication adherence and blood pressure control. *Journal of General Internal Medicine.* 2014;29(7):987–995.

38. Devine PG, Forscher PS, Austin AJ, Cox WTL. Long-term reduction in implicit race bias: a prejudice habit-breaking intervention. *Journal of Experimental Social Psychology.* 2012;48(6):1267–1278.

39. Blair IV. An investigation of associations between clinicians' ethnic or racial bias and hypertension treatment, medication adherence and blood pressure control. *Journal of General Internal Medicine.* 2014;29(7):987–995.

40. Hausmann LRM. Examining implicit bias of physicians who care for individuals with spinal cord injury: a pilot study and future directions. *The Journal of Spinal Cord Medicine.* 2015;38(1):102–110.

41. Hahn H, Aron LY, Lou C, Pratt E, Okoli A. Why does cash assistance depend on where you live? Washington, DC: Urban Institute. June 5, 2017. Available at: http://www.urban.org /research/publication/why-does-cash-welfare-depend-where-you-live.

42. Joy M, Clement T, Sisti D. The ethics of behavioral health information technology: frequent flyer icons and implicit bias. *JAMA*. 2016;316(15):1539–1540.

43. Buchs S, Mulitalo K. Implicit bias: an opportunity for physician assistants to mindfully reduce health care disparities. *The Journal of Physician Assistant Education*. 2016;27(4):193–195.

44. Kenison TC, Madu A, Krupat E, Ticona L, Vargas IM, Green AR. Through the veil of language: exploring the hidden curriculum for the care of patients with limited English proficiency. *Academic Medicine*. 2017;92:92–100.

45. Devine PG, Forscher PS, Austin AJ, Cox WTL. Long-term reduction in implicit race bias: a prejudice habit-breaking intervention. *Journal of Experimental Social Psychology*. 2012;48(6):1267–1278.

46. Zestcott CA, Blair IV, Stone J. Examining the presence, consequences, and reduction of implicit bias in health care: a narrative review. *Group Processes and Intergroup Relations*. 2016;19(4): 528–542.

47. Buchs S, Mulitalo K. Implicit bias: an opportunity for physician assistants to mindfully reduce health care disparities. *The Journal of Physician Assistant Education*. 2016;27(4):193–195.

48. Viswanathan V, Seigerman M, Manning E, Aysola J. Examining provider bias in health care through implicit bias rounds. *Health Affairs Blog*; July 17, 2017. Available at: http://healthaffairs .org/blog/2017/07/17/examining-provider-bias-in-health-care-through-implicit-bias-rounds/.

49. Sabin JA. The influence of implicit bias on treatment recommendations for 4 common pediatric conditions: pain, urinary tract infection, attention deficit hyperactivity disorder, and asthma. *American Journal of Public Health*. 2012;102(5):988–995.

Health Disparities and Their Structural Underpinnings

Part II of this text includes two chapters providing readers with an overview of the population health disparities in the United States and the ways in which these disparities are perpetuated by social and structural factors. Chapter 3 presents the history, trends, and epidemiology of health disparities for specific populations in the U.S. and explores some of their root causes. Chapter 4 describes social and structural factors that lead to population health inequity.

CHAPTER 3

Population Health Disparities

LEARNING OBJECTIVES

By the end of this chapter you will be able to:

- Define "population health disparities" and "vulnerable populations."
- Describe the history, trends, and epidemiology of health disparities for specific populations in the United States.
- Explain some of the root causes of health disparities, including the role of laws and policies in shaping these disparities.

▶ Introduction

In the Introduction to this text, we outlined a definition of *health equity* and how it may be distinguished from *health inequality, health disparity,* and *health care disparity*. We also presented a definition of *health justice* as "policies and societal behaviors that are evenhanded with regard to and display genuine respect for *everyone's* health and well-being." In this chapter, we contextualize these definitions by further exploring the history, trends, and epidemiology of health disparities by population group (e.g., by socioeconomic status, race, and gender). But in addition to presenting data and trend information about different types of health disparities in the United States, we explore the question, "Why do these disparities exist?" In the last 10 years, research on health disparities has evolved from describing differences in health among populations, to an attempt to understand *why* those differences exist and *how* they might be reduced or eliminated. See **FIGURE 3.1**.

Through the lens of health justice, this chapter describes some of the current understanding about the root causes of health disparities in the U.S. Other chapters (the chapters on existing safety net programs and legal protections and creating holistic systems to care for socially complex patients and populations) will explore and analyze some of the interventions, including laws and policies, which influence health disparities and may serve to either promote or undermine health equity. As you read

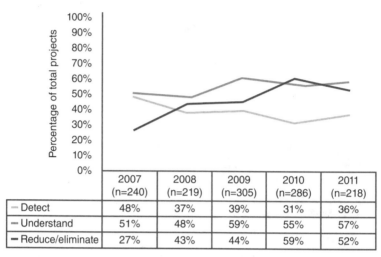

	2007 (n=240)	2008 (n=219)	2009 (n=305)	2010 (n=286)	2011 (n=218)
— Detect	48%	37%	39%	31%	36%
— Understand	51%	48%	59%	55%	57%
— Reduce/eliminate	27%	43%	44%	59%	52%

* Generation codes not mutually exclusive

FIGURE 3.1   Health equity research "generation" of disparities-focused health services research (2007–2011) n = 1,268.

Reproduced from Association of American Medical Colleges, The State of Health Equity Research: Closing Gaps to Address Inequities. 2014.

this chapter, ask yourself these questions: How have the discrete history, culture, and policy of the U.S. shaped the health disparities described? What structural changes, including laws, policies and system redesign, would promote health justice?

▶ Individual versus Population Health Disparities

Before we dive into specific types of health disparities, let's start with some more working definitions. First, what do we mean by *health*? The World Health Organization (WHO) offers a definition that has been widely accepted by public health professionals: "health is a state of complete physical, mental and social well-being and not merely the absence of disease or infirmity."[1] This definition implies that health is not simply a function of a person's genetic makeup, but that it is shaped and defined by social context. Accordingly, when measuring health disparities, researchers are not focused on differences in health between individuals, but rather differences by population group. Populations may be defined by many different characteristics—e.g., people in a certain age group, people living in a certain zip code, or people of a particular ethnic group. A widely cited definition of population health is that coined by David Kindig in 2007: "the distribution of health outcomes within a population, the determinants that influence distribution, and the policies and interventions that affect the determinants."[2] Notice that this definition implicates the role of policy in determining differences in population health.

▶ Vulnerable Populations

In our exploration of health disparities, we will focus on *vulnerable populations*. Kevin Grumbach and colleagues note that the word "vulnerable" comes from the Latin word for wounded: "in a sense, medically vulnerable populations are those that are wounded by social forces placing them at a disadvantage for their health."[3] Professors Mechanic and Tanner further define vulnerability as "an interaction between the capacities of individuals, the stresses that they are exposed to, and their various social networks, which can facilitate or hinder the ability of the individual to cope with various health challenges."[4] Below, we focus on the following vulnerable groups with documented health disparities: low socioeconomic status (SES) individuals, racial and ethnic minorities, immigrants, women, LGBT individuals, people with disabilities (including mental health and substance use disorders), people enmeshed with the criminal justice system, and rural populations. This is not an exhaustive list of groups who are vulnerable or susceptible to health disparities. We have selected these groups because the research provides strong evidence of health disparities in these populations.

It is important to keep in mind, as we explore different categories of vulnerability, that for many individuals, disparities may be overlapping. For example, low-SES people are more likely to be disabled; ethnic and racial minorities are more likely to be poor; and health care outcomes for women can vary based on race, ethnicity, and SES. As discussed above, health disparities are measured at the population level and often are described through a narrow focus on one type of vulnerability. Nonetheless, understanding how different kinds of vulnerability may overlap to create health disparities for individuals and groups is critical. As you read, think about the pathways between vulnerability and poor health and the ways in which multiple types of vulnerability may be at play in health disparities.

▶ Socioeconomic Status

When thinking about socioeconomic status (SES), people most often focus on income differences. But in fact, SES encompasses one's education, occupation, and income as they connect to social status or standing in relation to others. SES as an important determinant of health was first uncovered in the 1960s by a research team led by Michael Marmot, a British physician and epidemiologist, in longitudinal studies known as the "Whitehall Studies." What Dr. Marmot and his team discovered was that, despite universal access to health care through the National Health Service in the United Kingdom, health outcomes varied significantly by SES. Specifically, Marmot tracked health outcomes by differences in employment grade in the British civil service as a marker for social class, finding that "the lower a participant's status in his or her work hierarchy, the worse his or her health."[5] For example, for coronary heart disease, the researchers found that men in the lowest civil service grade were 3.6 times more likely to die from the disease than men in the highest grade. The differences persisted even after adjusting for health and lifestyle factors.[6]

What was truly groundbreaking in the Whitehall Studies is that researchers found a social gradient in health, meaning that the differences in health outcomes were not only present when comparing the highest and the lowest classes; they were present at every step of the social hierarchy. Marmot explains: "Socioeconomic differences in health are not confined to poor health for those at the bottom and good health for everyone else. Rather, there is a social gradient in health in individuals who are not poor: the higher the social position, the better the health. I have labeled this 'the status syndrome.'"[7]

While Americans may prefer to view the U.S. as a classless society without the type of social hierarchy in the U.K., a number of studies show that the

U.S. actually lags behind other countries in social mobility—the ability to move from the lower class to the middle class or from the middle class to upper class. A study by the Economic Mobility Project of the Pew Charitable Trusts found that 66% of Americans who started out in families in the top fifth for income remain in the top two-fifths, while 66% of those born in the bottom fifth stay in the bottom two-fifths.[8] Additionally, research on SES and health in the U.S. shows that a social gradient in health holds true, like that described by Marmot in the U.K. For example, a study of multiple health indicators for children and adults by SES found that: "those with the lowest income and who were least educated were consistently least healthy, but for most indicators, even groups with intermediate income and education levels were less healthy than the wealthiest and most educated."[9] SES is associated with a range of diseases, including low birthweight, hypertension, diabetes, cardiovascular disease, arthritis, and cancer. Low SES is also correlated with higher mortality.[10]

Understanding the pathways between SES and health is complex. What is the role of education versus income versus occupation? How do these factors influence one another? How do they independently or collectively influence health? In the chapter on social and structural barriers to health, we will explore each of these elements of SES and the roles (sometimes overlapping) that they seem to play in health disparities. However, understanding the role of SES in health goes beyond an understanding of a person's education level, occupation, or income. Marmot's research suggests that one's social status plays an important role well beyond material well-being. He points to one of the elements included in the WHO's definition of health: social well-being. Marmot explains:

> For people above the threshold of material well-being, another kind of well-being is central. Autonomy—how much control you have over your life—and the opportunities you have for full social engagement and participation are crucial for health, well-being, and longevity. It is inequality in these that plays a big part in producing social gradients in health. Degrees of control and participation underlie status syndrome.[11]

Another aspect of the role of social status in health is the notion of social capital. Ichiro Kawachi defines social capital as "those features of social relationships—such as levels of interpersonal trust and norms of reciprocity and mutual aid—that facilitate collective action for mutual benefit."[12] In a study of the relationship between social capital and health, Kawachi and his colleagues found that perceptions of trust in other people in one's community were correlated with death rates from heart disease, cancer, and infant mortality.[13] Social capital is closely connected to social inequality in a given community: living in a community with greater social inequality negatively influences perceptions of that community and the forces at play in the community, such as high levels of violence and social anxiety as well as increased perceptions of discrimination. "The combination of increasing social status differentials and the deteriorating social relations could hardly be a more potent mix for population health."[14] Social hierarchy, therefore, influences health at multiple levels. In the chapter on existing safety net programs and legal protections, we will further explore some of the mechanisms responsible for the links between SES and health. Now, we turn to a persistent problem in America: health disparities by race and ethnicity.

▶ Race and Ethnicity

As discussed above, health disparities are measured at the population level by categorizing individuals into groups based on a particular characteristic. Before describing disparities by race and ethnicity, we first need to explore how race has been used as a category in public health research. Consider the following statement by a member of the Institute of Medicine (IOM) Committee on Cancer Research Among Minorities and the Medically Underserved from 1999:

> The IOM committee recommends an emphasis on ethnic groups rather than on race in NIH's [National Institute of Health's] cancer surveillance and other population research. This implies a shift away from the emphasis on fundamental biological differences among "racial groups" to an appreciation of the range of cultural and behavioral attitudes, beliefs, lifestyle patterns, diet, environmental living conditions and other factors that may affect cancer risk.[15]

By shifting the classification from race to ethnicity, the committee was attempting to move away from notions of race as a biological or genetic construct to one that is social. The U.S. has a disturbing history with regard to racial classification that is infused with notions of white superiority. As such, race is an "inadequate and even harmful way to think about human biological differences."[16] From a scientific perspective, racial taxonomy is inadequate because: "(1) the concept of race is based on the idea of fixed, ideal, and unchanging types; (2) human variation is continuous; (3) human variation is nonconcordant [traits tend to vary independently of other traits; for example, 'skin color correlates with only a few other phenotypic traits such as hair and eye color']; (4) within-group genetic variation is much greater than variation among 'races'; (5) there is no way to consistently classify by race; (6) there is no clarity as to what race is and what it is not."[17] As a social construct, race can be understood as the social interpretation of certain physical characteristics (such as skin color and hair texture) and how people are perceived and valued based on their physical traits. It also recognizes the specific historical, social, and political context in which "race" has been understood in the U.S.

Yet, if researchers no longer use "race" as a category by which to understand health disparities, there is a danger of "minimizing the health impact of racism, especially for populations subjected to social prejudice because of their dark skin and facial features."[18] Race, in fact, is a powerful social category in the fight for health justice. As discussed below, research shows that the experience of racial discrimination itself may play a role in health disparities. In his book *The Death Gap*, Dr. David Ansell suggests:

> To think about race as a political classification requires us to redirect our causal explanations for racial inequities from the biological to the political structures of governance and social control that drive the inequities. If diseases are just biological events occurring within a person, then they require treatments directed only at the individual. But if we believe that racism and poverty cause diseases and premature mortality, then the solutions have to be directed at the economic systems and political structures that are perpetuating them.[19]

Because of the historical, political, and social significance of race in American society, researchers continue to try to parse out how the social experience of being categorized as part of a particular racial or ethnic group—e.g., black, white, Hispanic, or Asian—influences risk factors for adverse health outcomes. As we explore racial and ethnic health disparities, think about the value of collecting data using racial classifications. Is this categorization useful for framing policy and public health interventions, or does it reinforce embedded and troubling notions of race as biology?

Blacks and other ethnic minorities (including Hispanics and Native Americans) have significantly worse health outcomes than whites on a number of measures of morbidity and mortality. See **FIGURE 3.2**. Consider these statistics:

- Blacks have higher rates of diabetes, hypertension, and heart disease than other groups. Nearly 15% of blacks have diabetes compared with 8% of whites.
- Asthma prevalence is also highest among blacks. Black children have a 260% higher emergency department visit rate, a 250% higher hospitalization rate, and a 500% higher death rate from asthma compared to white children.
- Fourteen percent of Hispanics have been diagnosed with diabetes compared with 8% of whites. They have higher rates of end-stage renal disease, caused by diabetes, and they are 50% more likely to die from diabetes as non-Hispanic whites.
- One in five Latinos reports not seeking medical care due to language barriers.
- The prevalence of overweight and obesity in American Indian and Alaska Native preschoolers, school-aged children, and adults is higher than that for any other population group.
- In general, American Indian and Alaska Native adults are 60% more likely to have a stroke than their white adult counterparts and American Indian and Alaska Native women have twice the rate of stroke than white women.[20]

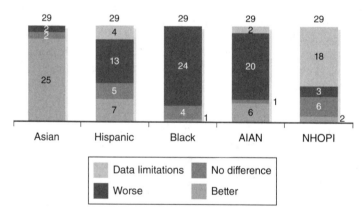

Note: Better or Worse indicates a statistically significant difference from white population at the p<0.05 level. No difference indicates there was no statistically significant difference. Data limitations indicates data are not available separately for a racial/ethnic group, insufficient data for a reliable estimate, or comparisons not possible to whites due to overlapping samples. AIAN refers to American Indians and Alaska Natives. NHOPI refers to Native Hawaiians and Other Pacific Islanders. Persons of Hispanic origin may be of any race but are categorized as Hispanic for this analysis; other groups are non-Hispanic.

FIGURE 3.2 Number of health status and outcome measures for which groups fared better, the same, or worse compared to whites.

The Henry J. Kaiser Family Foundation. Key Facts on Health and Health Care by Race and Ethnicity. June 7, 2016. http://www.kff.org/disparities-policy/report/key-facts-on-health-and-health-care-by-race-and-ethnicity/.

The difference in life expectancy between blacks and whites has narrowed in recent years, from 7 years in 1990 to 3.4 years in 2014. This narrowing may be in part due to so-called "deaths of despair," such as overdose deaths from the opioid crisis, which have affected more whites than blacks (this will be discussed in more detail later in this chapter). But it also may indicate a lowering in the death rate for blacks from cancer and cardiovascular disease.[21]

Nonetheless, researchers continue to explore why racial and ethnic health disparities persist. One explanation is that race and ethnicity serve as proxies for SES. Because race and ethnicity are strongly correlated with SES in the U.S., socioeconomic differences across racial and ethnic groups account for disparities in health status. "Researchers frequently find that adjusting racial disparities in health for SES substantially reduces these differences. In some cases the race disparity disappears altogether when adjusted for SES."[22] However, this is not always the case. In some studies, racial disparities persist at each level of SES. For example, infant mortality rates have been shown to be higher among college-educated black women than white college-educated peers.[23] This has led researchers to investigate other factors that may influence racial and ethnic health disparities. One theory offered by sociologist David Williams is that SES does not fully account for economic status differences. By focusing on educational attainment and income, but not wealth, measures of SES miss a part of the picture. Because there are large racial differences in the inheritance of and intergenerational transfer of wealth, SES does not fully capture economic disadvantage by race. He points out that net worth is significantly lower for blacks and Hispanics than for whites.[24]

Williams, as well as other researchers, point to another possible explanation: racism. As you will recall from the chapter on the effects of discrimination and implicit bias on health and health care, racism can operate at three levels, all of which may affect health: (1) interpersonal racism, or experiences of discrimination and prejudice experienced in everyday life; (2) internalized racism, in which victims of racism internalize prejudicial attitudes resulting in stress or loss of self-esteem; and (3) structural or institutionalized racism, which are "the structural elements of racism that are codified in our institutions of customs, practice and law so there need not be an identifiable perpetrator."[25] For individuals who experience discrimination, such as "everyday hassles of receiving poor service at restaurants, being followed or not helped in stores, and generally being treated with less respect and consideration than others,"[26] racism serves as a significant psychosocial stressor.

A number of studies have shown that the experience of racial discrimination is associated with poor health outcomes, including mental health disorders, hypertension, coronary artery disease, and poorer pregnancy outcomes.[27] As a *New York Times* article on the topic put it: "a growing body of evidence suggests that racial and sexual discrimination is toxic to the cells, organs and minds of those who experience it."[28] Because experiences of discrimination are internalized over the life course and can induce chronic stress, it may alter multiple body systems, leading to poor health outcomes. (We describe in more detail how chronic stress impacts body systems in the chapter on social and structural barriers to health).

One aspect of structural racism thought to have a significant effect on health outcomes is residential segregation. The legacy of racial segregation continues to track racial and ethnic minorities into neighborhoods with poor educational systems and lack of employment opportunities, perpetuating the intergenerational cycle of poverty. Living in a segregated neighborhood has been shown to negatively affect health as well as mortality rates.[29] For example, "health outcomes associated with residential segregation documented among black Americans include adverse birth outcomes, increased exposure to air pollutants, decreased longevity, increased risk of chronic disease, and increased rates of homicide and other crime."[30] **TABLE 3.1** provides a snapshot of some of the social, economic, and health inequities in the U.S. by race and ethnicity.

▶ Immigrant Status

In 2015, there were 43 million noncitizen immigrants living in the U.S., or roughly 13% of the population. Approximately 11 million immigrants residing in the U.S. are undocumented, meaning they have no legal status.[31] While rates of immigration have ebbed and flowed over time, the percentage of the U.S. population made up of immigrants has not significantly increased. See **FIGURE 3.3**. The top 10 countries of origin for immigrants in 2015 are presented in **FIGURE 3.4**.

The most common types of legal status are:

- Legal permanent residents ("green card" holders)
- Refugees (those living *outside* the U.S. seeking entry based on humanitarian reasons)
- Asylees (those living in the U.S. under temporary status, seeking permanent status based on humanitarian reasons)
- Those who have been granted temporary status, such as through the Deferred Action for Childhood Arrivals (DACA) program (for immigrants who were brought to the U.S. as children) or the Temporary Protected Status program (which, for example, covered Haitians after their country's earthquake in 2006)

Immigration status plays a large role in determining access to health care and other public services. Simply being legally present in the U.S. does not guarantee immediate access to all government-sponsored programs and services. For example, legal permanent residents must live in the U.S. five years before they can become eligible for Medicaid, a government-sponsored health insurance program for low-income and disabled individuals. In the chapter on existing safety net programs and legal protections, we describe in more detail how immigration status affects access to health insurance and health care. Here, we focus on the health status of immigrants in the U.S. as they compare to the native-born population.

Obviously, "immigrants" cannot be lumped into a single category for purposes of describing health disparities. As indicated above, they come from many different countries and have varied experiences in their home countries as well as in the U.S. Nevertheless, there are common health issues that are more frequently faced by immigrants and refugees, depending on country of origin, socioeconomic status, and access to resources. These include: mental health issues such as depression and post-traumatic stress disorder (often seen in refugees), tuberculosis, nutritional deficiencies and anemia, chronic hepatitis B, lack of immunization, and diabetes. At the same time, researchers have discovered the "immigrant paradox." That is, new immigrants actually have better health profiles than their native-born counterparts. However, the longer that an immigrant resides in the U.S., the more his or her health advantage declines over time.[32] Research suggests that, while the effect of the immigrant paradox varies among immigrant groups, it is most consistent among

TABLE 3.1 Social and Health Inequities in the U.S.

	Total	White non-Hispanic	Asian*	Hispanic or Latino	Black non-Hispanic[†]	Native American or Alaska Native
Wealth: median household assets (2011)	$68 828	$110 500	$89 339	$7683	$6314	NR
Poverty: proportion living below poverty level, all ages (2014); children <18 years (2014)	14.8%; 21.0%	10.1%; 12.0%	12.0%; 12.0%	23.6%; 32.0%	26.2%; 38.0%	28.3%; 35.0%
Unemployment rate (2014)	6.2%	5.3%	5.0%	7.4%	11.3%	11.3%
Incarceration: male inmates per 100 000 (2008)	982	610	185	836	3611	1573
Proportion with no health insurance, age <65 years (2014)	13.3%	13.3%	10.8%	25.5%	13.7%	28.3%
Infant mortality per 1000 live births (2013)	6.0	5.1	4.1	5.0	10.8	7.6
Self-assessed health status (age-adjusted): proportion with fair or poor health (2014)	8.9%	8.3%	7.3%	12.2%	13.6%	14.1%

(continues)

TABLE 3.1 Social and Health Inequities in the U.S. *(continued)*

	Total	White non-Hispanic	Asian*	Hispanic or Latino	Black non-Hispanic[†]	Native American or Alaska Native
Potential life lost: person-years per 100 000 before the age of 75 years (2014)	6621.1	6659.4	2954.4	4676.8	9490.6	6954.0
Proportion reporting serious psychological distress[‡] in the past 30 days, age ≥18 years, age-adjusted (2013–2014)	3.4%	3.4%	3.5%	1.9%	4.5%	5.4%
Life expectancy at birth (2014), years	78.8	79.0	NR	81.8	75.6	NR
Diabetes-related mortality: age-adjusted mortality per 100 000 (2014)	20.9	19.3	15.0	25.1	37.3	31.3
Mortality related to heart disease: age-adjusted mortality per 100 000 (2014)	167.0	165.9	86.1	116.0	206.3	119.1

NR = not reported. *Economic data and data on self-reported health and psychological distress are for Asians only; all other health data reported combine Asians and Pacific Islanders. [†]Wealth, poverty, and potential life lost before the age of 75 years are reported for the black population only; all other data are for the black non-Hispanic population. Serious psychological distress in the past 30 days among adults aged 18 years and older is measured using the Kessler 6 scale (range = 0–24; serious psychological distress: ≥13). Sources: Wealth data taken from the US Census; poverty data for adults taken from the National Center for Health Statistics; and poverty data for children taken from the National Center for Education Statistics; unemployment data taken from the US Bureau of Labor Statistics; incarceration data taken from the Kaiser Family Foundation; data on uninsured individuals taken from the National Center for Health Statistics; data on infant mortality, self-assessed health status, potential life lost, serious psychological distress, life expectancy, diabetes-related mortality, and mortality related to heart disease taken from the National Center for Health Statistics.

Reproduced from Bailey ZD, Krieger N, Agénor M, Graves J, Linos N, Bassett MT. Structural racism and health inequities in the USA: evidence and interventions. *Lancet*. April 8, 2017;389:1453–1463.

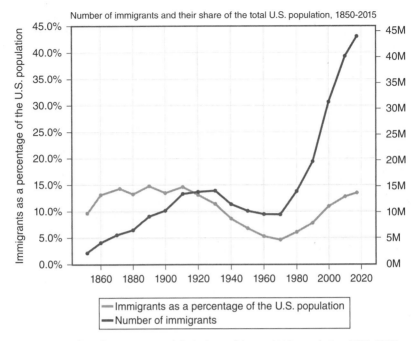

FIGURE 3.3 Number of immigrants and their share of the total U.S. population, 1850–2015.
Reproduced with permission from Migration Policy Institute.

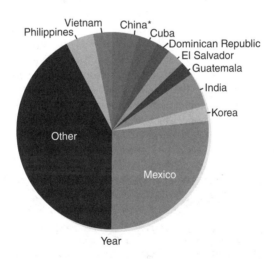

* The figure for China excludes both Hong Kong and Taiwan (1990-2016).

FIGURE 3.4 Top 10 largest immigrant groups, 2015.
Reproduced with permission from Migration Policy Institute.

Hispanic immigrants.[33] Researchers speculate that the decline in health over time is a function of acculturation—i.e., the adoption of an American lifestyle, including relatively high-calorie diets and sedentary lifestyles—leading to worsening health over time, and over generations, for immigrants and their families.

Immigrants experience a number of unique barriers to accessing health care in the U.S. See **FIGURE 3.5**. Many of these obstacles can lead to underutilization of health care by immigrants. Indeed, regardless of their legal status or insurance coverage, immigrants are less likely to receive preventive care than citizens.[34] Delayed care can mean that when immigrants do seek care (often in an emergency department), they present sicker and have more complex health care needs because of untreated chronic illness.

Immigrants who are undocumented may be particularly reluctant to seek health care, fearing that they may be reported to authorities. One study in North Carolina found that: "among immigrant Hispanics/Latinos, the fear of deportation, a lack of required forms of documentation, interaction with law enforcement personnel, and racial profiling are factors also associated with reduced utilization of health services and worse health."[35] These fears have only been exacerbated in recent years with political and media attention to stepped up immigration enforcement efforts. Additionally, because undocumented immigrants are not eligible for Medicaid or Medicare, or for financial assistance in the purchasing of health insurance under the Affordable Care Act, they may forgo care altogether due to the cost. In fact, all immigrants, regardless of status, are less likely to be insured than citizens. See **FIGURE 3.6**.

As described above, however, insurance access is only one of the barriers to health care for immigrants. Language barriers present a particularly difficult obstacle for many immigrants in seeking health care and understanding diagnoses and treatment regimens. While there are protections under federal civil rights laws (specifically, Title VI of the 1964 Civil Rights Act) requiring health systems to provide adequate language interpretation services to ensure that appropriate care is provided to non-English speaking patients, many systems are underresourced and thus do not provide adequate services. Studies suggest that language barriers can have a significant impact on health care quality and treatment. For example, one study showed that Latino children living in households with non-English primary language "have a significantly higher odds of perforation of the appendix than non-Latino children in English primary language households.[36] Access to quality, appropriate health care for immigrants is determined by laws and policies governing eligibility for government programs, including public health insurance. But the health of immigrants in the U.S. is also strongly influenced by how health system resources are allocated and removal of health system barriers to care.

Barriers to health care for immigrants

- Limited English proficiency
- Fear, especially among undocumented patients
- Ineligibility for public benefits
- Discrimination
- Distrust of large institutions
- No preventive care in country of origin
- Different understanding of causes of/remedies to illness
- Complexity of U.S. health insurance systems
- Lack of transportation

FIGURE 3.5 Barriers to health care for immigrants.

Data from Morton S, Sprecher M, Shuster L, Cohen E. Legal status: meeting the needs of immigrants in the health care setting. In: Tobin Tyler E, et al. *Poverty, Health and Law: Readings and Cases for Medical-Legal Partnership*. Durham: Carolina Academic Press; 2012: 317.

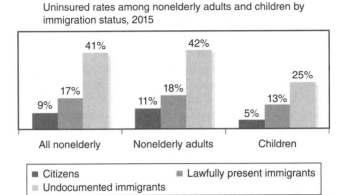

Uninsured rates among nonelderly adults and children by immigration status, 2015

Note: All non-citizen percentages shown are statistically significantly different from the respective citizen percentage at the p<0.05 level.

FIGURE 3.6 Uninsured rates among nonelderly adults and children by immigration status, 2015.

The Henry J. Kaiser Family Foundation, Health Coverage and Care for Immigrants. July 11, 2017. https://www.kff.org/disparities-policy /issue-brief/health-coverage-and-care-for-immigrants/.

▶ Gender

In general, women may be viewed as having better health than men. After all, they enjoy a longer life expectancy than men—eight years longer. But women's unique experiences, including their social, economic, and political position in society and their greater role in reproduction make them a vulnerable population that experiences particular health disparities. In fact, life expectancy for lower-educated women, particularly white women, actually has declined in recent years.[37]

Furthermore, while women are less likely to die at each age than men, they are more likely to rate their health as poor and to visit the hospital more than men. This paradox may be explained, at least in part, by differences in the prevalence of chronic conditions women face. Women experience higher rates of pain (headaches, arthritis), and some respiratory conditions, including bronchitis, asthma, and lung problems not related to cancer. They are also much more likely to suffer from reproductive cancers, hypertension, vision problems, and depression [than men].[38]

On the other hand, earlier mortality for men may be tied to riskier unhealthy behaviors. "Their higher rates of cigarette smoking, heavy drinking, gun use, employment in hazardous occupations, and risk taking in recreation and driving are responsible for males' higher death rate due to lung cancer, accidents, suicide, and homicide."[39]

It is difficult to sort out the factors that influence gender differences in morbidity and mortality. While biological factors, including hormonal influences, play a role, environmental, cultural, and social factors also clearly impact health behaviors and outcomes. Some of the key factors influencing women's health are that they are more likely to be poor and to work in low-wage jobs, often despite having better educational credentials, and to raise children on their own. In the U.S., poverty is highest in households headed by single women, among women of color, and for elderly women living alone. One in three single-mother families are poor, and one in eight women overall are poor.[40] As explored in detail in the chapter on social and structural barriers to health, poverty is strongly correlated with a range of poor health outcomes. This is particularly the case for stress-related conditions, such as depression, anxiety, diabetes, hypertension, obesity, and arthritis, and thus perhaps it is not surprising that women tend to suffer from these conditions in greater numbers than men. Another is violence. While men are more likely than women to die from homicide and suicide, women are also more likely to be the victims of intimate partner violence, with one in five women experiencing it during their lifetime. (Intimate partner violence is also discussed in greater detail in the chapter on social and structural barriers to health.)

Data on women's health also illustrate significant racial and ethnic health disparities. These include higher rates of diabetes for black and Latina women, and higher-risk pregnancies for black women may represent higher rates of low SES for women of color. Black women are also at significantly higher risk of contracting human immunodeficiency virus (HIV) and of dying from acquired immunodeficiency syndrome (AIDS)—they account for nearly half of new infections and deaths from HIV/AIDS. Public health officials posit that this disparity may result from the higher incarceration rate for black men, who infect their female partners.[41] They also have higher mortality rates from heart disease, stroke, and cancer. One explanation for the higher mortality rates from these diseases for black women is lower screening rates and worse access to preventive services.[42]

The World Health Organization (WHO) reports that worldwide, women are twice as likely as men to experience depression, and depression may also be more persistent for women than for men. The WHO notes that: "gender specific risk factors for common mental disorders that disproportionately affect women include gender based violence, socioeconomic disadvantage, low income and income inequality, low or subordinate social status and rank and unremitting responsibility for the care of others."[43] Women are more likely to seek help for mood disorders, such as depression and anxiety than are men, and more likely to be prescribed psychotropic medications.[44]

Women also experience barriers to health care. As of 2015, roughly 11% of women ages 19 to 64, or about 11 million women, were uninsured.[45] Lack of health insurance significantly affects the quality of care that women receive. Uninsured women are less likely to access preventive services such as mammograms and Pap tests and to have a regular source of care, including prenatal care. Women of color, immigrant women, and low-income women are most likely to be uninsured, as are single mothers.[46] At least, however, the Affordable Care Act (ACA) prohibits gender-rating insurance (meaning that health insurance plans cannot charge women more than men for the same benefits) and requires that ACA plans cover certain preventive services without a copayment, including well women visits, Pap tests, mammograms, bone density tests, the human papilloma virus (HPV) vaccine, breastfeeding supplies, and prescription contraceptives. Clearly an effort to expand and improve women's access to care—especially preventive services that are particular important to women's health—the ACA made great strides in reducing inequity in women's health care.

However, due to political controversy, the drafters of the ACA compromised with opponents by not including coverage for abortion services. Furthermore, ongoing controversy over the ACA's contraceptive mandate has led to lawsuits (discussed in the chapter on existing safety net programs and legal protections) and threats from the Trump Administration to eliminate the mandate. Women's health, and particularly women's reproductive health, continues to be subject to social, economic, and political forces. These forces affect women's daily lives: "[b]ecause so much of women's lives is devoted to reproductive issues—trying to avoid pregnancy, trying to get pregnant, raising children, and being familial caretakers—women are directly affected by the politicization of reproductive health care."[47]

▶ Sexual Orientation and Gender Identity (Lesbian, Gay, Bisexual, and Transgender Health)

In addition to gender-based health disparities between men and women, sexuality and gender identity–based health disparities are important to consider in a health justice framework. Individuals who identify as lesbian, gay, bisexual, and/or transgender (LGBT) have distinct health concerns, many of which derive from discrimination, stigma, and lack of access to health care that is responsive to their particular needs. The Centers for Disease Control and Prevention (CDC) reports that 1.8% of men self-identify as gay and 0.4% identify as bisexual, while 1.5% of women self-identify as lesbian and 0.9% identify as bisexual.[48] According to one study, 1.4 million people identify as transgender.[49] Accurate estimates of LGBT people in the U.S. are difficult to come by, however, since they rely on self-identification and because stigma may lead to underreporting.

Until recently, research on health disparities associated with being LGBT has been limited. "The generalizability of many early studies was limited by their techniques, such as nonrandom enrollment methods, lack of heterosexual controls, low response rates, and over-representation of white and educated subjects."[50] The AIDS epidemic in the 1980s heightened recognition of the particular health risks associated with being LGBT, which include higher rates of obesity, tobacco and substance use, mental health issues, injury and violence, and difficulty accessing appropriate health care. Lesbians, in particular, have a higher prevalence of overweight and obesity than heterosexual women, which puts them at risk for other health problems, such as cardiovascular disease and diabetes. They are also at higher risk for breast and ovarian cancer, perhaps due to later childbearing, less oral contraceptive use, and obesity.[51] Lesbians may also be less likely to seek routine cancer screenings due to feeling stigmatized by the medical care system.[52] In addition, hormone use may increase the risk of cardiovascular disease in transgender patients. Gay and bisexual men, particularly young black men, remain at heightened risk for HIV.[53] It is also important to note that the growing research on the negative effects of stigma, discrimination, and stress on health, including both physical and mental health, is applicable to the LGBT population as well as other minority groups discussed above.

Of significant concern for the LGBT population are mental health disorders, particularly depression and anxiety. These disorders are "not inherent to being a sexual minority person but can manifest as a result of leading marginalized lives, enduring the stress of hiding one's sexuality, or facing verbal, emotional, or physical abuse from intolerant family members and communities."[54] A recent study comparing transgender and nontransgender individuals found that transgender identity was associated with higher risk for reported discrimination, depression, and attempted suicide. Self-acceptance of transgender identity was correlated with lower rates of reported depression.[55] LGBT adolescents are at increased risk of suicidal ideation, as well as for homelessness.[56]

Until 1973, homosexuality was included as a mental health disorder in the *Diagnostic and Statistical Manual of Mental Disorders*, which is published by the American Psychiatric Association and offers standard criteria for the classification of mental disorders. The legacy of stigmatizing sexual minorities as mentally ill or deviant from the norm has shaped the LGBT community's relationship with the health care system, creating significant barriers to trusting provider-patient relationships. In addition, permissible discrimination against LGBT people in employment, housing, and, until recently, marriage laws has affected health and access to care. For example, until the U.S. Supreme Court decided in the 2015 case of *Obergefell v. Hodges* that same-sex couples have a constitutional right to marry,[57] these couples could not access spousal benefits through employer-sponsored health insurance. While strides have been made in recent years in securing more legal protections for LGBT people, health and health care inequities remain a concern, especially for transgender people.

Research on the health and health care needs of LGBT people is relatively new and needs development to improve access to appropriate care. The Institute of Medicine (IOM) Committee on Lesbian, Gay, Bisexual, and Transgender Health Issues and Research Gaps and Opportunities identified the need for multifactorial research and strategies to improve the health and health care access of the LGBT community. The Committee noted that the LGBT community is not monolithic and that the health and health care needs of gay men, lesbians, bisexuals, and transgender individuals should be studied independently, but that understanding the intersectionality within this population is also important[58] (see **FIGURE 3.7**). The health

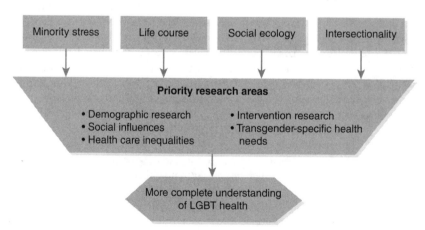

FIGURE 3.7 Research agenda for LGBT health issues.

Data from Institute of Medicine (US) Committee on Lesbian, Gay, Bisexual, and Transgender Health Issues and Research Gaps and Opportunities. Summary. The health of lesbian, gay, bisexual, and transgender people: building a foundation for better understanding. Washington, DC: National Academies Press; 2011. https://www.ncbi.nlm.nih.gov/books/NBK64795/.

and health care needs of the LBGT population is perhaps the most politicized area of health equity policy. There is still not even agreement among policymakers and health care providers that services should be provided that recognize the particular experiences and needs of this population.

▶ Disability

People with disabilities are often not recognized as a population for which there are health disparities. The medical model "treats disability as a problem of the person, directly caused by disease, trauma or other health condition, which requires medical care."[59] This model assumes that health differences for people with disabilities are individual. But, as we have discussed, health disparities are not just health differences; they are closely connected to social and economic disadvantage. The "social model" recognizes that "disability is not an attribute of the individual, but rather a complex collection of conditions which are created by the social environment."[60] The International Classification of Functioning Disability and Health (ICF), published by the World Health Organization in 2001, makes clear that "disability" is not simply a biomedical label, but rather should be understood in social and environmental context:

> In the ICF framework, disability is used as an umbrella term to include bodily impairments, activity limitations, or participation restrictions that relate to a health condition. These limitations, which interact with personal and contextual factors of the environment, result in disability. That is, a disability results from the interaction of having a condition-based limitation and experiencing barriers in the environment.[61]

The U.S. Department of Health and Human Services' *Healthy People 2020*, an initiative which sets 10-year goals and objectives for improving population health, has embraced the social understanding of disability, recognizing "that what defines individuals with disabilities, their abilities, and their health outcomes more often depends on their community, including social and environmental circumstances."[62] Because research surveys use different definitions of disability, prevalence data varies. The 2010 U.S. Census, which uses the American Community Survey and asks about six types of difficulties associated with disability—hearing, vision, cognitive, ambulatory, self-care, and independent living—reveals that 19% of Americans—nearly one in five—have a disability.[63]

Historically, discrimination and social barriers have it made it difficult for people with disabilities to find employment, have equal educational opportunities, and to participate in social life, all of which are correlated with good health. While laws such as the Americans with Disabilities Act and the Individuals with Disabilities Education Act have greatly improved employment and educational opportunity for people with disabilities, they still struggle with employment and educational barriers, which in turn may lead to lower socioeconomic status, which is strongly associated with poor health. People with disabilities also experience barriers in access to health care and other health promoting activities and services, such as opportunities for physical fitness. People with disabilities have an increased risk of chronic disease such as hypertension, obesity, and depression, are more likely to smoke, are less likely to get adequate physical activity, and are less likely to have social interactions.[64]

In addition to disability-related disparities, rates of disability vary across demographic groups: low-income Americans are much more likely to have a disability than those with higher income; blacks and Native Americans also have higher rates of disability than whites and Asians.[65] Minorities who are disabled experience greater disparities than adults who are minorities without disabilities or nonminorities with mobility limitations alone.[66] Data from the U.S. National Health Interview Survey show that "among the measures with the greatest disparities were worsening health, depressive symptoms, diabetes, stroke, visual impairment, difficulty with activities of daily living, obesity, physical activity and low workforce participation."[67]

People with mental illness and those with substance use disorders also experience significant disparities in access to health care. Individuals with serious mental illness are more likely to die from chronic disease than those without mental illness. Drug dependence is considered a mental illness, "because addiction changes the brain in fundamental ways, disturbing a person's normal hierarchy of needs and desires and substituting new priorities connected with procuring and using the drug. The resulting compulsive behaviors that override the ability to control impulses despite the consequences are similar to hallmarks of other mental illnesses."[68] Some people with mental illness and/or drug dependence may be considered disabled if their disorder impairs their daily functioning. Stigma associated with mental illness may exacerbate the development of comorbid chronic disease, particularly because of the strong association between mental illness, homelessness, and poverty.

Research has documented considerable health care disparities for people with disabilities. Adults with mobility limitations are less likely than nondisabled adults to receive preventive screenings for cholesterol or blood pressure checks, even though they have higher rates of high cholesterol and high blood pressure. Women with mobility limitations are also more likely to experience late-stage breast cancer detection. Children with disabilities are less likely to have regular dental care.[69] Lack of training of health care providers about the particular health determinants and health care needs of people with disabilities compounds these access issues. For individuals with mental illness, access to care may be significantly undermined when primary care providers are not adequately prepared to respond to mental health problems as part of medical care. Integration of mental health services into primary care— discussed in the chapter on creating holistic systems to care for socially complex patients and populations—is a promising model of care delivery that may help to remove some of these barriers to appropriate care.

Another obstacle to care for people with disabilities is the role that health care providers play in determining if a patient qualifies for Social Security Disability benefits. Under the law, physicians must apply a legal definition of "disability" set by the Social Security Administration, which essentially asks the physician to judge whether or not the patient can "engage in substantial gainful activity"[70] based on medically proven sensory, physical, or mental impairments. While critically important to the patient's well-being, this process can sometimes disrupt the provider-patient relationship if care becomes focused on determining whether the patient qualifies for disability benefits rather than the broader health needs of the patient. Improving health and health care for people with disabilities requires a multipronged approach that recognizes the social, environmental, economic, and health system factors that contribute to their health. See **BOX 3.1**.

BOX 3.1 WHO Principles of Action Recommendations

The WHO Principles of Action recommends the following to achieve health equity among individuals with disabilities:

1. Improving the conditions of daily life by:
   - Encouraging communities to be accessible so all can live in, move through, and interact with their environment
   - Encouraging community living
   - Removing barriers in the environment using both physical universal design concepts and operational policy shifts
2. Addressing the inequitable distribution of resources among individuals with disabilities and those without disabilities by increasing:
   - Appropriate health care for individuals with disabilities
   - Education and work opportunities
   - Social participation
   - Access to needed technologies and assistive supports
3. Expanding the knowledge base and raising awareness about determinants of health for individuals with disabilities by increasing:
   - The inclusion of individuals with disabilities in public health data collection efforts across the lifespan
   - The inclusion of individuals with disabilities in health promotion activities
   - The expansion of disability and health training opportunities for public health and health care professionals.[70]

World Health Organization (WHO), Commission on Determinants of Health. Closing the gap in a generation: health equity through action on the determinants of health. Final report. Geneva, Switzerland: WHO; 2008.

▶ Incarceration

Recall from the Introduction to this text that the U.S. has an incarceration rate that exceeds that of every other nation in the world. As a refresher, review the following two graphs (**FIGURE 3.8** and **FIGURE 3.9**), which highlight incarceration trends over time and incarceration rates by race and ethnicity.

Incarceration itself has a profound effect on the health of individuals and communities. It also represents the ways in which multiple layers of disadvantage overlap to perpetuate health, racial, social, and economic inequity. People who are or have been incarcerated are disproportionately poor, undereducated, uninsured, homeless, and racial minorities compared to the general population.[71] They bear a much higher burden of disease and disability than their nonincarcerated counterparts. In addition to higher rates of mental illness and substance use disorders, they also have a higher prevalence of chronic and infectious diseases. HIV is approximately four times higher in correctional settings than in the general population; hepatitis C virus (HCV) is nine to ten times higher. Incarcerated individuals also have higher rates of sexually transmitted diseases and tuberculosis when compared with the general public.[72] The incarcerated are also more likely to have disabilities. More than one-third of prison inmates suffer from at least one disability (not including substance use disorders), including 19.5% of prisoners who have developmental or intellectual disabilities.[73] Incarcerated individuals are four to six times more likely than the general public to report Down syndrome, autism, dementia, learning disorders, and intellectual disabilities.[74]

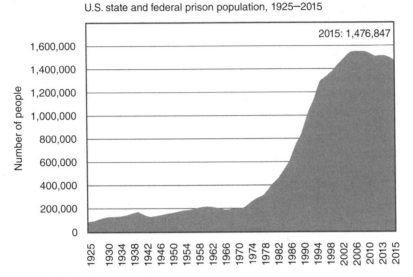

FIGURE 3.8 Trends in U.S. corrections.

The Sentencing Project. U.S. State and Federal Prison Population, 1925–2015. Fact Sheet: Trends in U.S. corrections.
http://sentencingproject.org/wp-content/uploads/2016/01/Trends-in-US-Corrections.pdf.

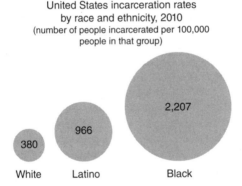

FIGURE 3.9 United States incarceration rates by race and ethnicity, 2010.

Data from Prison Policy Initiative. United States incarceration rates by race and ethnicity, 2010. https://www.prisonpolicy.org/graphs/raceinc.html.

Many of the diseases and disabilities prevalent in the incarcerated population—mental illness, substance use, HIV, and cognitive disabilities—carry significant stigma. Coupling this stigma with that of poverty, homelessness, and incarceration intensifies health disparities and social inequality. The overlapping disadvantage and stigma experienced by incarcerated individuals does not end with discharge from prison or jail. So called "collateral consequences" play an important role in disadvantage as well. These are "the penalties and disabilities that occur automatically as a result of conviction, apart from the sentence itself. These include a whole host of disadvantages: disenfranchisement; ineligibility for public benefits, housing, scholarships and student loans; loss of occupational licenses, employment and child custody; and felon registration requirements."[75] Sixty-five million people in the U.S. have a criminal record,[76] and the collateral consequences they suffer perpetuate poverty, unemployment, homelessness, and food insecurity, all key social determinants of health. They also reinforce stigma and social exclusion, which are also important contributors to poor health.[77]

In addition to the health disparities experienced by incarcerated individuals, mass incarceration has perpetuated health disparities in families of the incarcerated and in communities with high rates of criminal justice involvement. Children who have an incarcerated parent are susceptible to feelings of shame and stigma and are at higher risk for stress-related illness. Women with incarcerated partners are also at increased risk for social isolation and depression.[78] While there has not been significant research completed on the effects of incarceration on community health, it is known that incarceration is not evenly divided across communities, and some studies suggest that the experience of living in a community with high rates of incarceration may impact health. One study found that individuals who report having a friend or family member incarcerated in the past five years also report worse health overall, along with more mental health problems and stress.[79] The family and community disruption created by incarceration, as well as the collateral consequences that create significant barriers for incarcerated individuals upon reentry into their communities, not only undermine that individual's success; they also significantly destabilize social cohesion in the community.

Prior to passage of the Affordable Care Act, access to affordable health insurance was unavailable for most low-income single adults. Thus, most incarcerated individuals were likely to have been uninsured. Without insurance, many in this population had no regular source of primary care or access to mental health and substance use services prior to incarceration. A study of jail inmates undertaken prior to ACA passage found that 80% of jail inmates with chronic health problems did not receive regular medical care prior to incarceration, and 90% did not have health insurance.[80] The ACA's expansion of Medicaid to low-income single adults made it possible for this population to access health insurance, often for the first time. However, because the ACA's Medicaid expansion is optional for states, individuals who live in states that did not adopt the expansion still have no access to affordable health insurance, and likely no regular source of health care.

Ironically, the first time many incarcerated individuals receive primary health care is while in prison. In 1976, the Supreme Court held in *Estelle v. Gamble* that the provision of health care is mandated in correctional facilities, since incarcerated individuals are effectively wards of the state and unable to seek need care on their own.[81] However, a review of prison health care concludes that: "it appears clear . . . that actual medical treatment is consistently provided for only a fraction of those needing it, whether for HIV, chronic conditions, mental health, or substance abuse."[82] The health and health care disparities experienced by the incarcerated and formerly incarcerated populations demonstrate the confluence of social, health, and criminal justice policy and their overlapping effects on health. To be sure, American "hyperincarceration," particularly of low-income, undereducated black men, has exacerbated longstanding racial health disparities in black communities.

▶ Rural Populations

While we often associate poverty-based health disparities with urban communities, the U.S. rural population is overall more likely to live in poverty than populations living in metropolitan areas. A quarter of the rural population has incomes below the federal poverty level, compared to one-fifth of the population living in metropolitan areas.[83] Furthermore, while there has been a loss of manufacturing jobs and subsequent rising rates of unemployment in rural areas, urban America has experienced population and economic growth, as well as expanded health care and public health initiatives focused on addressing chronic disease.[84] Rural communities experience a higher burden of heart disease, stroke, diabetes, tobacco use, substance abuse, and mental health disorders than metropolitan areas. They also have a much higher prevalence of injury-related deaths: there is a 22% higher risk of injury-related death in rural communities and more than half of all car accident fatalities occur in rural areas.[85]

Recent research has focused on rural health outcomes and has sought answers to why they seem to be worsening. A widely cited 2015 study by Anne Case and Angus Deaton, describing the rising mortality rates among whites ages 45 to 54 with a high school education or less, points to the growth in "deaths of despair"—deaths from drug and alcohol poisonings, suicide, and chronic liver diseases and cirrhosis. They note that: "self-reported declines in health, mental health, and ability to conduct activities of daily living and increases in chronic pain and inability to work, as well as clinically measured deteriorations in liver function, all point to growing distress in this population."[86] A 2017 study that examined causes of death by subpopulation found that "in addition to deaths from suicide, accidental poisoning, and liver disease, Whites in rural areas saw increases in chronic disease deaths, which contributed to the overall higher increases in death rates in these subpopulations."[87] While the opioid crisis and rising mortality rates has raised awareness about poor health in white rural communities, some have cautioned against losing focus on persistent racial health disparities:

> We should guard against the unintended consequence that the focus on the increase in death rates in some Whites (significant as they are) detract attention from the persistent health inequities by race and social class, which are so large that they dwarf the size of what is a very troublesome increase in some Whites. The fact that the despair explanation has been so quickly adopted (with personal responsibility explanations being quickly discarded) to explain the mortality increase in Whites, despite persistent questioning of the relevance of factors like despair to Black–White differences, is itself telling. It raises interesting questions about how causal explanations emerge and what influences the speed with which they are adopted.[88]

While diseases of despair may explain rising mortality rates in rural communities, many point to persistent disparities in access to health care as a critical factor in the health of rural populations, as well. People living in rural communities may have more limited access to health insurance, and they are less likely to be covered by employer-sponsored insurance than the metropolitan population. They are also less likely to have access to Medicaid, despite the high rates of poverty in rural areas. Nearly two-thirds of the rural uninsured live in states that did not expand Medicaid to single adults under the Affordable Care Act. Consequently, rural people are much more likely (15%) than their urban counterparts (9%) to fall into the "coverage gap," meaning that their income is too low for them to qualify for financial assistance to purchase private insurance, which was designed to help more moderate-income people.[89]

Rural areas also suffer from significant shortages of health care providers. Rural communities have roughly 40 physicians per 100,000 people, while urban areas have 53 per 100,000 people. Access to care in rural areas is also hindered by the greater distances individuals must travel to see a provider. This can be especially true with regard to specialists.[90] Interestingly, some studies suggest that the more limited number of primary care providers may actually serve to make continuity of care stronger in rural communities. But there may be ramifications to the lack of access to health care in rural communities. Studies show that rural patients are also less likely to receive screening and diagnostic testing, including cancer screenings, compared with patients in urban areas.[91] **TABLE 3.2** provides a snapshot of some of the health and health care issues in rural communities.

One of the most chronic shortages in rural communities is that of mental health providers. This shortage, combined with heightened stigma around mental health care in rural communities, creates significant barriers for rural populations.[92] Given the prevalence of mental health disorders in these communities, this remains a major concern for improving health and well-being in rural America.

TABLE 3.2 National Health Snapshot: Rural and Urban

National Rural Health Snapshot	Rural	Urban
Percentage of population	19.3%	80.7%
Number of physicians per 10,000 people	13.1	31.2
Number of specialists per 100,000 people	30	263
Population aged 65 and older	18%	12%
Average per capita income	$45,482	$53,657
Non-Hispanic white population	69–82%	45%
Adults who describe health status as fair/poor	19.5%	15.6%
Adolescents who smoke	11%	5%
Male life expectancy in years	76.2	74.1
Female life expectancy	81.3	79.7
Percentage of dual-eligible Medicare beneficiaries	30%	70%
Medicare beneficiaries without drug coverage	16%	13%
Percentage covered by Medicaid	43%	27%

All information in this table is from the Health Resources and Services Administration and Rural Health Information Hub.

Reproduced from National Rural Health Association. About rural health care, https://www.ruralhealthweb.org/about-nrha/about-rural-health-care

▶ Conclusion

This chapter explored health disparities in the U.S. through the lens of health justice. This approach entailed stepping back and first considering how people are classified for purposes of studying populations and examining some of the historical and social contexts in which these classifications were derived, particularly with regard to race. The study of health disparities is not a study of the biological differences among individuals, but a study of the social and political underpinnings that shape which groups are more likely to suffer from poor health than others. Parsing out the multiple factors that influence health and health disparities can be complex. Yet, as we have seen, social status, stigma, and access to resources clearly play a large role in health justice. In the next chapter, we turn to specific social and structural factors and their effect on population health, particularly for the most vulnerable populations described here.

References

1. World Health Organization. Constitution of World Health Organization: Principles. Available at: www.who.int/about/mission/en/.
2. Kindig DA. Understanding population health terminology. *Milbank Quarterly.* 2007;85(1):139–161.
3. Grumbach K, Braveman P, Adler N, Bindman AB. Vulnerable populations and health disparities: an overview. In: King TE, Wheeler MB, Bindman AB, et al., eds. *Medical Management of Vulnerable and Underserved Populations: Principles, Practice and Populations.* New York, NY: McGraw Hill; 2007: 3.
4. Mechanic D, Tanner J. Vulnerable people, groups, and populations: societal view. *Health Affairs.* 2007;26:1220–1230.
5. Goldberg D, Baxley EG, Fancher TL. Socioecologic determinants of health. *Health Systems Science.* AMA Education Consortium. 2017;134–152, 136.
6. Marmot MG, Rose G, Shipley M, Hamilton PJ. Employment grade and coronary heart disease in British civil servants. *Journal of Epidemiology and Community Health.* 1978;32(4):244–249.
7. Marmot, M. Status syndrome: a challenge to medicine. *JAMA.* 2006;295:1304–1307.
8. The Pew Charitable Trusts Economic Mobility Project. Pursuing the American dream: economic mobility across generations; July 2012. Available at: http://www.pewtrusts.org/~/media/legacy/uploadedfiles/pcs_assets/2012/pursuingamericandreampdf.pdf.
9. Braveman PA, Cubbin C, Egerter S, Williams DR, Pamuk E. Socioeconomic disparities in health in the United States: what the patterns tell us. *American Journal of Public Health.* April 2010;100(Suppl 1):S186–S196.
10. Adler NE, Newman K. Socioeconomic disparities in health: pathways and policies. *Health Affairs.* March 2002;21(2):60–76.
11. Marmot M. *The Status Syndrome: How Social Status Affects Our Health and Longevity.* New York, NY: Henry Holt; 2004.
12. Kawachi, I. Social capital and community effects on population and individual death. *Annals of the New York Academy of Sciences.* 1999;896:120–130, 121.
13. Kawachi, I. Social capital and community effects on population and individual death. *Annals of the New York Academy of Sciences.* 1999;896:120–130, 121.
14. Wilkinson, RG. Health, hierarchy, and social anxiety. *Annals of the New York Academy of Sciences.* 1999;896:48–63, 50.
15. Haynes MA, Smedley BD, eds. *The Unequal Burden of Cancer: An Assessment of NIH Research and Programs for Ethnic Minorities and the Medically Underserved.* Washington, DC: National Academies Press; 1999.
16. Goodman, AL. Why genes don't count (for differences in health). In: LaVeist TA, Isaac LA, eds. *Race, Ethnicity, and Health: A Public Health Reader,* 2nd ed. San Francisco, CA: Jossey-Bass; 2013: 50–53.

17. Goodman, AL. Why genes don't count (for differences in health). In: LaVeist TA, Isaac LA, eds. *Race, Ethnicity, and Health: A Public Health Reader,* 2nd ed. San Francisco, CA: Jossey-Bass; 2013: 50–53.

18. Thomas, SB. The color line: race matters in the elimination of health disparities. In: LaVeist TA, Isaac LA, eds. *Race, Ethnicity, and Health: A Public Health Reader,* 2nd ed. San Francisco, CA: Jossey-Bass; 2013: 36.

19. Ansell D. *The Death Gap: How Inequality Kills.* Chicago, IL: University of Chicago Press; 2017: 62.

20. Center for American Progress. Fact sheet: health disparities by race and ethnicity; December 16, 2010. Available at: https://www.americanprogress.org/issues/healthcare/news/2010/12/16/8762/fact-sheet-health-disparities-by-race-and-ethnicity/. Accessed October 9, 2017.

21. Stein EM, Gennuso KP, Ugboaja DC, Remington PL. The epidemic of despair among white Americans: trends in the leading causes of premature death, 1999–2015. *American Journal of Public Health.* October 2017;107(10):1541–1547.

22. Williams DR, Collins C. U.S. socioeconomic and racial differences in health. In: LaVeist TA, Isaac LA, eds. *Race, Ethnicity, and Health: A Public Health Reader,* 2nd ed. San Francisco, CA: Jossey-Bass; 2013: 36.

23. Williams DR, Collins C. U.S. socioeconomic and racial differences in health. In: LaVeist TA, Isaac LA, eds. *Race, Ethnicity, and Health: A Public Health Reader,* 2nd ed. San Francisco, CA: Jossey-Bass; 2013: 36.

24. Williams DR, Collins C. U.S. socioeconomic and racial differences in health. In: LaVeist TA, Isaac LA, eds. *Race, Ethnicity, and Health: A Public Health Reader,* 2nd ed. San Francisco, CA: Jossey-Bass; 2013: 36.

25. Grumbach K, Braveman P, Adler N, Bindman AB. Vulnerable populations and health disparities: an overview. In: King TE, Wheeler MB, Bindman AB, et al., eds. *Medical Management of Vulnerable and Underserved Populations: Principles, Practice and Populations.* New York, NY: McGraw Hill; 2007.

26. Bailey ZD, Krieger N, Agénor M, Graves J, Linos N, Bassett MT. Structural racism and health inequities in the USA: evidence and interventions. *Lancet.* April 8, 2017;389:1453–1463, 1457.

27. Williams DR, Mohammed SA. Racism and health I: pathways and scientific evidence. *The American Behavioral Scientist.* 2013;57(8):1152–1173; Williams DR, Neighbors HW, Jackson JS. Racial/ethnic discrimination and health: findings from community studies. *American Journal of Public Health.* 2003;93(2):200–208.

28. Khullar D. How prejudice can harm your health. *The New York Times.* June 8, 2017. Available at: https://www.nytimes.com/2017/06/08/upshot/how-prejudice-can-harm-your-health.html?mcubz=1 (citing recent research on discrimination and health).

29. Williams DR, Collins C. U.S. socioeconomic and racial differences in health. In: LaVeist TA, Isaac LA, eds. *Race, Ethnicity, and Health: A Public Health Reader,* 2nd ed. San Francisco, CA: Jossey-Bass; 2013: 36.

30. Bailey ZD, Krieger N, Agénor M, Graves J, Linos N, Bassett MT. Structural racism and health inequities in the USA: evidence and interventions. *Lancet.* April 8, 2017;389:1453–1463, 1457.

31. Migration Policy Institute. Frequently requested statistics on immigrants and immigration in the United States; March 8, 2017. Available at: http://www.migrationpolicy.org/article/frequently-requested-statistics-immigrants-and-immigration-united-states#CurrentHistoricalNumbers. Accessed October 9, 2017.

32. Williams, DR. The health of US racial and ethnic populations. *Journals of Gerontology Series.* 2005;60B(11):53–62, 56.

33. Mendoza FS. Health disparities and children in immigrant families: a research agenda. *Pediatrics.* November 2009;124(Supp. 3):S187–S195.

34. Morton S, Sprecher M, Shuster L, Cohen E. Legal status: meeting the needs of immigrants in the health care setting. In: Tobin Tyler E, et al., eds. *Poverty, Health and Law: Readings and Cases for Medical-Legal Partnership.* Durham, NC: Carolina Academic Press; 2012: 317.

35. Rhodes SD, Mann L, Simán FM, et al., The impact of local immigration enforcement policies on the health of immigrant Hispanics/Latinos in the United States. *American Journal of Public Health.* February 2015;105(2):329–337.

36. Flores G. Families facing language barriers in healthcare: when will policy catch up with the demographics and evidence? *Journal of Pediatrics.* June 2014;164(6):1261–1264.

37. Montez JK, Zajacova A. Why is life expectancy declining among low-educated women in the United States? *American Journal of Public Health.* 2014;104(10):e5–e7.

38. Population Reference Bureau. Gender disparities in health and mortality, Available at: http://www.prb.org/Publications/Articles/2007/genderdisparities.aspx. Accessed October 9, 2017.

39. Population Reference Bureau. Gender disparities in health and mortality. Available at: http://www.prb.org/Publications/Articles/2007/genderdisparities.aspx. Accessed October 9, 2017.

40. National Women's Law Center. Data on poverty and income. Available at: https://nwlc.org/issue/data-on-poverty-income/. Accessed October 9, 2017.

41. Shrage L. Why are so many black women dying of AIDS? *The New York Times,* Opinion. December 11, 2015. Available at: https://www.nytimes.com/2015/12/12/opinion/why-are-so-many-black-women-dying-of-aids.html?_r=0.

42. Harleman E, Steinauer J. Women's health: reproduction and beyond in poor women. In: King TE, Wheeler MB, Bindman AB, et al. *Medical Management of Vulnerable and Underserved Populations: Principles, Practice and Populations.* New York, NY: McGraw Hill; 2007: 299–300.

43. World Health Organization. Gender disparities and mental health: the facts. Available at: http://www.who.int/mental_health/prevention/genderwomen/en/. Accessed October 9, 2017.

44. World Health Organization. Gender disparities and mental health: the facts. Available at: http://www.who.int/mental_health/prevention/genderwomen/en/. Accessed October 9, 2017.

45. The Henry J. Kaiser Family Foundation. Women's health insurance coverage fact sheet; October 21, 2016. Available at: https://www.kff.org/womens-health-policy/fact-sheet/womens-health-insurance-coverage-fact-sheet/. Accessed October 9, 2017.

46. The Henry J. Kaiser Family Foundation. Women's health insurance coverage fact sheet; October 21, 2016. Available at: https://www.kff.org/womens-health-policy/fact-sheet/womens-health-insurance-coverage-fact-sheet/. Accessed October 9, 2017.

47. Harleman E, Steinauer J. Women's health: reproduction and beyond in poor women. In: King TE, Wheeler MB, Bindman AB, et al. *Medical Management of Vulnerable and Underserved Populations: Principles, Practice and Populations.* New York, NY: McGraw Hill; 2007: 297.

48. Ward BW, Dahlhamer JM, Galinsky AM, Joestl SS. Sexual orientation and health among U.S. adults: National Health Interview Survey; 2013. Atlanta, GA: Centers for Disease Control and Prevention, National Center for Health Statistics. Available at: https://www.cdc.gov/nchs/data/nhsr/nhsr077.pdf.

49. Flores AR, Herman JL, Gates GJ, Brown TNT. How many adults identify as transgender in the United States? Los Angeles, CA: The Williams Institute; June 2016. Available at: http://williamsinstitute.law.ucla.edu/wp-content/uploads/How-Many-Adults-Identify-as-Transgender-in-the-United-States.pdf.

50. Rosenthal A, Diamant A. Sexuality as vulnerability: the care of lesbian and gay patients. In: King TE, Wheeler MB, Bindman AB, et al. *Medical Management of Vulnerable and Underserved Populations: Principles, Practice and Populations.* New York, NY: McGraw Hill; 2007: 275.

51. Rosenthal A, Diamant A. Sexuality as vulnerability: the care of lesbian and gay patients. In: King TE, Wheeler MB, Bindman AB, et al. *Medical Management of Vulnerable and Underserved Populations: Principles, Practice and Populations.* New York, NY: McGraw Hill; 2007: 275.

52. Mayer KH, Bradford JB, Makadon HJ, Stall R, Goldhammer H, Landers S. Sexual and gender minority health: what we know and what needs to be done. *American Journal of Public Health.* June 2008;98(6):989–995.

53. Institute of Medicine (US) Committee on Lesbian, Gay, Bisexual, and Transgender Health Issues and Research Gaps and Opportunities. Summary. The health of lesbian, gay, bisexual, and transgender people: building a foundation for better understanding. Washington, DC: National Academies Press; 2011. Available at https://www.ncbi.nlm.nih.gov/books/NBK64795/. Accessed October 9, 2017.

54. Mayer KH, Bradford JB, Makadon HJ, Stall R, Goldhammer H, Landers S. Sexual and gender minority health: what we know and what needs to be done. *American Journal of Public Health.* June 2008;98(6):989–995.

55. Su D, Irwin JA, Fisher C, Ramos A. Mental health disparities within the LGBT population: a comparison between transgender and nontransgender individuals. *Transgender Health.* 2016;1(1):12–20.

56. Institute of Medicine (US) Committee on Lesbian, Gay, Bisexual, and Transgender Health Issues and Research Gaps and Opportunities. Summary. The health of lesbian, gay, bisexual, and transgender people: building a foundation for better understanding. Washington, DC: National Academies Press; 2011. Available at https://www.ncbi.nlm.nih.gov/books /NBK64795/. Accessed October 9, 2017.

57. Obergefell v. Hodges, 135 S. Ct. 2584 (2015).

58. Institute of Medicine (US) Committee on Lesbian, Gay, Bisexual, and Transgender Health Issues and Research Gaps and Opportunities. Summary. The health of lesbian, gay, bisexual, and transgender people: building a foundation for better understanding. Washington, DC: National Academies Press; 2011. Available at https://www.ncbi.nlm.nih.gov/books /NBK64795/. Accessed October 9, 2017.

59. Kushel M, Iezzoni LI. Disability and patients with disability. In: King TE, Wheeler MB, Bindman AB, et al. *Medical Management of Vulnerable and Underserved Populations: Principles, Practice and Populations.* New York, NY: McGraw Hill; 2007: 384.

60. Kushel, M, Iezzoni LI. Disability and patients with disability. In: King TE, Wheeler MB, Bindman AB, et al. *Medical Management of Vulnerable and Underserved Populations: Principles, Practice and Populations.* New York, NY: McGraw Hill; 2007: 384.

61. Krahn GL, Walker DK, Correa-De-Araujo R. Persons with disabilities as an unrecognized health disparity population. *American Journal of Public Health.* 2015;105(S2):S198–S206, S198.

62. U.S. Department of Health and Human Services. *Healthy People 2020.* Disability and health overview. Available at: https://www.healthypeople.gov/2020/topics-objectives/topic /disability-and-health. Accessed October 9, 2017.

63. U.S. Census Bureau. Survey of income and program participation, June–September 2005 and May–August 2010, Table 1. Prevalence of disability for selected age groups: 2005 and 2010. Available at https://www.census.gov/people/disability/publications/disab10/table_1.pdf.

64. U.S. Department of Health and Human Services. *Healthy People 2020.* Disability and health overview. Available at: https://www.healthypeople.gov/2020/topics-objectives/topic /disability-and-health. Accessed October 9, 2017.

65. American Association on Health and Disability. Health disparities and people with disabilities; March 2011. Available at: https://www.aahd.us/wp-content/uploads/2012/03 /HealthDisparities2011.pdf.

66. American Association on Health and Disability. Health disparities and people with disabilities; March 2011. Available at: https://www.aahd.us/wp-content/uploads/2012/03 /HealthDisparities2011.pdf.

67. American Association on Health and Disability. Health disparities and people with disabilities; March 2011. Available at: https://www.aahd.us/wp-content/uploads/2012/03 /HealthDisparities2011.pdf.

68. U.S. Department of Health and Human Services, National Institute on Drug Abuse. Comorbidity: addiction and other mental illnesses; September 2010. Available at: https:// www.drugabuse.gov/sites/default/files/rrcomorbidity.pdf.

69. American Association on Health and Disability. Health disparities and people with disabilities; March 2011. Available at: https://www.aahd.us/wp-content/uploads/2012/03 /HealthDisparities2011.pdf.

70. Social Security Administration. Definition of Disability. Available at: https:www.ssa.gov /disability/professionals/bluebook/general-info.htm.

71. Western B, Pettit B. Incarceration and social inequality. *Daedalus: Journal of the American Academy of Arts and Sciences.* Summer 2010.

72. Rich JD, Wohl DA, Beckwith CG, et al. HIV-related research in correctional populations: now is the time. *Current HIV/AIDS Reports.* 2011;8(4):288–296, 289–290; Varan AK, Mercer DW, Stein MS, Spaulding AC. Hepatitis C seroprevalence among prison inmates since 2001: still high but declining. *Public Health Reports.* 2014;129(2):187–195.

73. Mizrahi J, Jeffers J, Ellis EB, Pauli P. Disability and criminal justice reform: keys to success. RespectAbilityUSA. Available at: https://www.respectability.org/wp-content/uploads/2017/05 /Disability-and-Criminal-Justice-Reform-White-Paper.pdf. Accessed October 9, 2017.

74. Vallas R. Disabled behind bars: the mass incarceration of people with disabilities in America's jails and prisons. Center for American Progress; 2016: 2.

75. Tobin Tyler E, Brockmann B. Returning home: incarceration, reentry, stigma and the perpetuation of racial and socioeconomic health inequity. *Journal of Law, Medicine & Ethics* 2017;45(4):545–557.

76. Garretson HJ. Legislating forgiveness: a study of post-conviction certificates as policy to address the employment consequences of a conviction. *Public Interest Law Journal.* 2016;15:1–41.

77. Tobin Tyler E, Brockmann B. Returning home: incarceration, reentry, stigma and the perpetuation of racial and socioeconomic health inequity. *Journal of Law, Medicine & Ethics* 2017;45(4):545–557.

78. Schnittker J, Massoglia M, Uggen C. Incarceration and the health of the African American community. *Du Bois Review.* 2011;8:1–9.

79. Kruger DJ, Hill De Loney E. The association of incarceration with community health and racial health disparities. *Progress in Community Health Partnerships: Research, Education and Action.* 2009;3(2):113–121, 113.

80. Patel K, Boutwell A, Brockmann BW, Rich JD. Integrating correctional and community health care for formerly incarcerated people who are eligible for Medicaid. *Health Affairs.* 2014;33(3):468–473, 469.

81. Estelle v. Gamble, 429 U.S. 97 (1976).

82. Dumont DM, Allen SA, Brockmann BW, et al. Incarceration, community health, and racial disparities. *Journal of Health Care for the Poor and Underserved.* February 2013;24(1):78–88, 83.

83. The Henry J. Kaiser Foundation. The Affordable Care Act and insurance coverage in rural areas. May 29, 2014. Available at: https://www.kff.org/uninsured/issue-brief/the-affordable -care-act-and-insurance-coverage-in-rural-areas/. Accessed October 9, 2017.

84. Stein EM, Gennuso KP, Ugboaja DC, Remington PL. The epidemic of despair among white Americans: trends in the leading causes of premature death, 1999–2015. *American Journal of Public Health.* October 2017;107(10):1541–1547.

85. National Rural Health Association. About rural health. Available at: https://www .ruralhealthweb.org/about-nrha/about-rural-health-care. Accessed October 9, 2017.

86. Case A, Deaton A. Rising morbidity and mortality in midlife among white non-Hispanic Americans in the 21st century. *Proceedings of the National Academy of Sciences.* 2015; 112(49):15078–15083. Available at: http://www.pnas.org/content/112/49/15078. Accessed October 9, 2017.

87. Stein EM, Gennuso KP, Ugboaja DC, Remington PL. The epidemic of despair among white Americans: trends in the leading causes of premature death, 1999–2015. *American Journal of Public Health.* October 2017;107(10):1541–1547.

88. Diez Roux AV. Despair as a cause of death: more complex than it first appears. Editorial. *American Journal of Public Health.* October 2017;107(10):1566–1567.

89. The Henry J. Kaiser Foundation. The Affordable Care Act and insurance coverage in rural areas. May 29, 2014. Available at: https://www.kff.org/uninsured/issue-brief/the-affordable -care-act-and-insurance-coverage-in-rural-areas/. Accessed October 9, 2017.

90. Spoont M, Greer N, Su J, et al. Rural vs. urban ambulatory health care: a systematic review [Internet]. Washington, DC: U.S. Department of Veterans Affairs; May 2011. Summary and discussion. Available at: https://www.ncbi.nlm.nih.gov/books/NBK56140/. Accessed October 9, 2017.

91. Spoont M, Greer N, Su J, et al. Rural vs. urban ambulatory health care: a systematic review [Internet]. Washington, DC: U.S. Department of Veterans Affairs; May 2011. Summary and discussion. Available at: https://www.ncbi.nlm.nih.gov/books/NBK56140/. Accessed October 9, 2017.

92. Spoont M, Greer N, Su J, et al. Rural vs. urban ambulatory health care: a systematic review [Internet]. Washington, DC: U.S. Department of Veterans Affairs; May 2011. Summary and discussion. Available at: https://www.ncbi.nlm.nih.gov/books/NBK56140/. Accessed October 9, 2017.

CHAPTER 4

Social and Structural Barriers to Health

LEARNING OBJECTIVES

By the end of this chapter you will be able to:

- Discuss the social and structural factors that affect population health and contribute to health disparities.
- Explain how unmet social needs contribute to specific health disparities.
- Describe how "toxic stress," resulting from social and environmental exposures, contributes to a number of chronic health conditions.

▶ Introduction

As described in the chapter on population health disparities, health disparities do not occur naturally; they are the result of complex pathways between our social environment and our biology. Each of us is born into a family that exists in a larger social, cultural, economic, and political environment that helps to shape our health (see **FIGURE 4.1**). In this chapter, we explore the social and structural factors that influence the distribution of health. As you read, think about how different social and structural barriers affect the health of populations, and also how these barriers relate to and overlap with one another. Think further about the ways in which policies and systems could be redesigned to improve health equity and promote health justice.

▶ The Growth of Income and Wealth Inequality in America

We start with the issue of income and wealth inequality because, as we will describe, income and wealth are highly correlated with health outcomes. Income inequality in America has been growing since the 1980s. While the incomes of the wealthiest

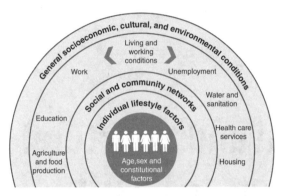

FIGURE 4.1 The social and structural determinants of health.

Dahlgren G, Whitehead M. Policies and strategies to promote social equity in health. Stockholm Institute for Future Studies; 1991.

1% of the population grew 192% from 1980 to 2015, incomes of those in the bottom 20% grew only 46% over the same period and the incomes of those in the middle 60% grew just 41% (see **FIGURE 4.2**). In addition to increasing income inequality, there has been a rising concentration of wealth at the top since the 1980s as well. Income is the money that a household earns over the course of a year. Wealth is a person's total net worth—assets (property, investments) minus any liabilities (debt). A 2014 report by the National Bureau of Economic Research found that the wealthiest 1% of households own 42% of the nation's wealth.[1] **FIGURE 4.3** shows that the bottom 90% own only a quarter of the country's wealth.

▶ Inequality and Poverty

As income and wealth inequality have grown, so too have health disparities between the rich and poor. In a landmark study of the relationship between income inequality and health, researchers Richard Wilkinson and Kate Pickett mapped countries by income inequality against an index of health and social problems, finding that the two are highly correlated. The United States, which has the highest level of income inequality among comparison nations, also measured worst on the index of health and social problems (see **FIGURE 4.4**).

The gap in life expectancy between the wealthiest and poorest Americans has been widening since the 1970s and is now 10 years for women and nearly 15 years for men.[2] As described in the chapter on population health disparities, health disparities research clearly demonstrates that socioeconomic status is a strong predictor of health. In fact, it is well established that health is distributed across a social gradient running from top to bottom of the social hierarchy, with those at the top having the best health, those at the bottom having the worst health, and those in middle having worse health than those above them and better health than those below them. In this section, we focus on those at the bottom of the social hierarchy and the large role that poverty plays in poor health. To understand why poverty is such an important predictor of health outcomes, we first explore some key questions about poverty itself: how is poverty defined and who is poor in America? After discussing poverty generally, we turn to the causes of poverty, its effects on health, and the role of unmet social needs in health disparities.

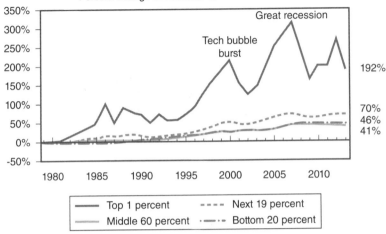

FIGURE 4.2 Income gains at the top dwarf those of low- and middle-income households.

Data from Center for Budget and Policy Priorities. A guide to statistics on historical trends in income inequality. December 5, 2013. http://dsodown.mywebtext.org/pdf/s06-Trends_Income_Inequality.pdf.

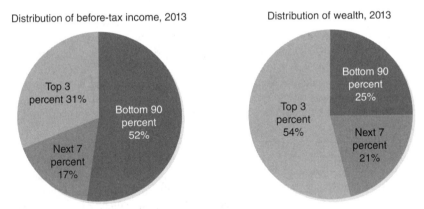

FIGURE 4.3 Wealth is even more concentrated than income.

Data from Center for Budget and Policy Priorities. A guide to statistics on historical trends in income inequality. December 5, 2013. http://dsodown.mywebtext.org/pdf/s06-Trends_Income_Inequality.pdf.

What Does It Mean to Be Poor in America?

In his book, *Poverty in America*, John Iceland defines poverty simply, as "economic, or income, deprivation," and describes two types of poverty measures—an *absolute* measure and a *relative* measure. Absolute poverty measures assume that there is a "measurable subsistence level of income or consumption below which people should be deemed economically disadvantaged or deprived," while relative measures are based on "the notion that poverty is relative to a society's existing level of economic, social and cultural development."[3] In other words, poverty is defined by comparative economic deprivation—one's status relative to others in his country, state, or

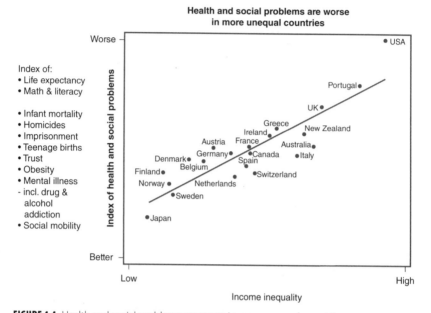

FIGURE 4.4 Health and social problems are worse in more unequal countries.

© Wilkinson R, Pickett, K., 2009, *The Spirit Level: Why Greater Equality Makes Societies Stronger.* New York: Bloomsbury Press, an imprint of Bloomsbury Publishing Inc.

local community. The United States tends to favor absolute measures of poverty.[3] For example, as will be described in the chapter on existing safety net programs and legal protections, most federal social safety net programs use a threshold income level—based on family size and regardless of changes to the family's standard of living—for purposes of program eligibility. At the same time, states sometimes use median household income—a relative measure of poverty—to determine eligibility for programs.

Defining who is poor using a relative measure implies that poverty may differ depending on the country in which one lives. In other words, it may be different to be poor in a wealthy nation like the U.S. than it is to be poor in a very low-income country, such as Bangladesh. It also raises interesting (and controversial) questions about what may be considered the "basic needs" of an individual or family living in the U.S. Is having access to a car a basic need in the U.S.? Can one have a cell phone and be considered poor? Does owning a washing machine, computer, or television, or having air conditioning imply that a family is not poor? What might be considered luxuries in other countries may seem like basic needs in the U.S., given the nation's relative overall wealth. Some argue that having items like cell phones and air conditioners means that a family should not be considered poor. As we explore what we call "social needs" and their relation to health below, think about these questions.

Who Is Poor in America?

Using official government measures of poverty, 46 million Americans were living in poverty in 2014. The majority of Americans living below the poverty level are children. A quarter of those living in poverty are in the labor force, with the disabled,

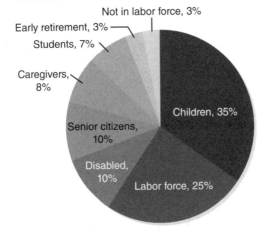

Characteristics of individuals living below poverty, 2014

FIGURE 4.5 Characteristics of individuals living below poverty, 2014.

Data from the Brookings Institution. Who is poor in America? June 17, 2016. https://www.brookings.edu/research/who-is-poor -in-the-united-states/.

senior citizens, and caregivers making up significant percentages of the poor. Refer to **FIGURE 4.5**.

Women are three times more likely to live in poverty than men; more than one in eight women and more than one in three single mothers are poor. Women of color are significantly more likely to live in poverty than white women: 23.1% of black, 22.7% of Native American, and 20.9% of Hispanic women live in poverty, as compared to 9.5% of white women and 7.1% of white men.[4]

▶ The Effects of Poverty on Health (and Health on Poverty)

While the causal pathways between poverty and health are complex, there are a number of theories that have been developed to explain them. First, poverty is not just a lack of income; it is associated with a range of other social conditions that may affect health—like access to quality education, health care, housing, nutritious food, and employment opportunities. Second, recent research shows that poverty is associated with higher levels of stress and that stress in childhood is highly correlated with poor long-term health outcomes. (This will be discussed in detail later in the chapter.) Third, poverty and health are connected bidirectionally. If one is poor, he or she is more likely to have health problems, but having health problems may also lead one to be poor. The inability to work due to illness or disability contributes to poverty.

To understand how poverty is associated with poor health, it is important to understand that poverty may encompass multiple social determinants of health and that these often influence one another. We explore the range of social factors that influence the health of low-income and vulnerable populations later in this chapter.

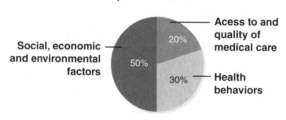

FIGURE 4.6 Social determinants of health.

Data from from the University of Wisconsin Population Health Institute's County Health Rankings model © 2010. htttp://www
.countyhealthrankings.org/about-project/background.

▶ Defining and Estimating Social and Structural Determinants of Health

The Centers for Disease Control and Prevention (CDC) define the social determinants of health as:

> The complex, integrated, and overlapping social structures and economic systems that are responsible for most health inequities. These social structures and economic systems include the social environment, physical environment, health services, and structural and societal factors. Social determinants of health are shaped by the distribution of money, power, and resources throughout local communities, nations, and the world.[5]

Researchers have attempted to estimate the significance of social and environmental factors in the health of individuals and populations. Most estimate that between 40% and 60% of health is attributable to social, environmental, and economic factors, while access to needed medical care accounts for only 10% to 20%.[6] See **FIGURE 4.6.**

The field of social epidemiology has made great strides in the past decade in pointing to the ways in which "social structures, institutions, and relationships influence health… and how societies are organized to produce or impede the development and maintenance of good health."[7] Social structures that affect population health may include how societies allocate resources—such as money for health care and education—through their tax system, and how societies structure government services and regulate private markets—including the design of food programs and the regulation of the housing, transportation, and real estate markets.

▶ Unmet Social Needs and Health

As our understanding of health has expanded to include the importance of non-medical and structural factors, researchers have pointed to the fact that the U.S. stands alone (among its peer nations) in allocating far more resources to medical care than it does to social services and supports. In fact, some argue that we have "medicalized" poverty and social problems rather than address them as root causes of poor health. While access to quality health care is critically important, it is but one social determinant of health and as described earlier, a relatively small contributor to a person's overall health. In focusing on access to medical care, policy has failed to move upstream to address the unmet social needs that contribute to poor health.

Researchers Elizabeth Bradley and Lauren Taylor have demonstrated that the U.S. is an outlier among its peer nations in outspending every other one on health care services, while significantly underspending for social services, such as education, housing, economic development, and job training. They found that nations in the Organisation for Economic Co-operation and Development (a forum made up of 34 countries with market-based economies who work together to promote economic growth and prosperity) spend two dollars on social services for every one dollar spent on health care—except for the U.S., which spends just fifty-five cents on social services for every dollar spent on health care. Bradley and Taylor also assessed how this difference in spending might affect health outcomes. Here, they found that countries, as well as some states, with a higher ratio of social service to healthcare spending have better health outcomes on many measures. They argue that better integration of medical and social services could improve health outcomes and reduce health disparities.[8] In the chapter on creating holistic systems to care for socially complex patients and populations, we describe some of the innovative models that are being implemented to better integrate medical and social services.

As you read below about the many social and structural determinants of health, consider what you think to be the most appropriate allocation of health and social care resources to most improve population health and reduce health disparities. We start by discussing access to health care as a determinant of health because, despite significant strides in reducing the number of people without health insurance, there are still many people in the U.S. who are uninsured, underinsured, and/or do not have access to regular health care.

▶ Access to Health Care

Because there is no legal right to health care nor a universal government-sponsored health insurance program, the U.S. has substantially higher rates of uninsured citizens than other comparable nations, many of which provide government-funded insurance (for core health services) to all citizens. For most low- and moderate-income Americans, the out-of-pocket costs for health care are prohibitively expensive, and thus having adequate insurance coverage for both preventive and catastrophic care is required to access needed health care services. Of course, having health insurance does not ensure access to appropriate quality health care, but it is the first step in making access to services possible for most Americans. The Patient Protection and Affordable Care Act of 2010 (ACA) expanded access to health insurance in two ways. First, it expanded eligibility for Medicaid, a federal public insurance program for the poor and disabled, which is primarily funded by the federal government and administered by states. The ACA expanded Medicaid coverage to all individuals below 138% of the federal poverty level. Second, the ACA created a mandate that all citizens acquire health insurance or pay a tax, providing subsidies to low- and moderate-income individuals to offset the cost of insurance premiums.

Since it was passed in 2010, the Affordable Care Act has dramatically reduced the number of uninsured, from roughly 50 million to 27 million people. From 2013 to 2015, there were significant reductions in the percentage of uninsured blacks (from 17% to 12%) and Latinos (from 25% to 17%).[9] Despite these gains, a large segment of the population remains uninsured. Because the U.S. Supreme Court determined that expansion of the Medicaid program under the ACA was optional, not required, for states, many of the poorest adults in states that did not expand Medicaid remain without coverage or a regular source of health care. It is well documented that the uninsured are less likely than those with insurance to have a regular source of primary care or to receive services for major health conditions, including chronic disease.[10] Given the high cost of health care, those without insurance are much more likely to go without care than the insured. Prior to the ACA, 39% of low- to moderate-income Americans reported not seeking care when they needed it due to cost.[11] Even for those who are able to obtain insurance, they may be underinsured, meaning that high deductibles, cost sharing, and/or inadequate or lack of coverage for certain services may prevent them from seeking and receiving care.

In addition to expanding Medicaid, the ACA also increased funding for community health centers that serve low-income and otherwise vulnerable populations. This has increased consumption of health care by the poorest Americans.[12] Overall, the law has reduced disparities in access to care in both states that expanded Medicaid and those that did not, with the greatest reductions in states that did.[13] Nonetheless, disparities in access to and utilization of health care persist for people of color (see **FIGURE 4.7**) and in the quality of care received by patients based on income (see **FIGURE 4.8**).

Historically, one of the major challenges of ensuring that low-income individuals have access to health care is that Medicaid's reimbursement rates to care providers are significantly lower than rates offered by Medicare (another federal insurance program, primarily for the elderly) and by private insurance carriers. This has led to a shortage of providers willing to accept Medicaid patients, which, in turn, has led to wait times for patient appointments. This is particularly true in rural areas where there are already fewer providers than in urban areas. Studies indicate that

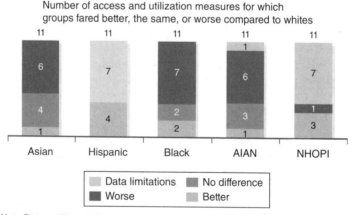

Note: Better or Worse indicates a statistically significant difference from White population at the p<0.05 level. No difference indicates there was no statistically significant difference. Data limitations indicates data are not available separately for a racial/ethnic group, insufficient data for a reliable estimate, or comparisons not possible to Whites due to overlapping samples. AIAN refers to American Indians and Alaska Natives. NHOPI refers to Native Hawaiians and Other Pacific Islanders. Persons of Hispanic origin may be of any race but are categorized as Hispanic for this analysis; other groups are non-Hispanic.

FIGURE 4.7 Number of access and utilization measures for which groups fare better, the same, or worse compared to whites.

The Henry J. Kaiser Family Foundation, Key Facts on Health and Health Care by Race and Ethnicity, June 2016. https://www.kff.org /disparities-policy/report/key-facts-on-health-and-health-care-by-race-and-ethnicity/.

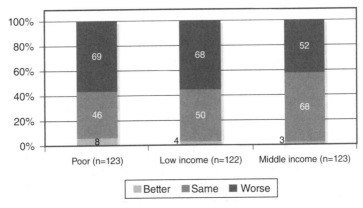

FIGURE 4.8 Number and percentage of all quality measures that were improving, not changing, or worsening, total and by priority area, from 2000 through 2014.

Agency for Healthcare Research and Quality, 2016 Healthcare Quality and Disparities Report. https://www.ahrq.gov/research/findings/nhqrdr/nhqdr16/quality.html.

since the ACA increased Medicaid reimbursement to payment levels used for the Medicare program, the availability of new primary care appointments has increased for Medicaid recipients.[14]

A critical question regarding access to insurance and to health care is: what is the effect of access on health outcomes? Does having insurance and better access to health care actually improve health? One study suggests that the answer is yes. Assessing the effects of Massachusetts' decisions to expand insurance coverage to near-universal levels and to expand access to care, the study found that the reforms in Massachusetts were associated with a significant decrease in deaths amenable to health care. This was particularly true in counties with lower household incomes and where there had been high uninsurance rates prior to the reform.[15] Massachusetts' reforms are widely viewed as the blueprint for the Affordable Care Act.

Because of the increases in chronic disease rates, particularly among low-income Americans, over the last several decades, access to health insurance and to a regular source of health care is important in reducing the burden of disease on the poor. Coverage expansions under the ACA could have significant benefits for chronic disease identification and management in populations who have heretofore lacked access to care.[16] But in addition to coverage expansions, access to a regular, high-quality source of preventive care for all Americans is needed to ensure that the health care system is fair and equitable.

▶ **Food and Nutrition**

Just as access to a regular, quality source of health care improves health outcomes, access to sufficient amounts of nutritious and affordable food is necessary for optimal health, including physiological, cognitive, and emotional functioning. Food insecurity in a household may be described as the following: "At times during the year, these households were uncertain of having, or unable to acquire, enough food to meet the needs of all their members because they had insufficient money or other resources for food."[17] The U.S. Department of Agriculture (USDA), which tracks food insecurity in the U.S., distinguishes between low food security and very low food security. *Low food security* is associated with "reports of reduced quality, variety, or desirability of diet but little or no indication of reduced food intake." *Very low food security* is associated with "reports of multiple indications of disrupted eating patterns and reduced food intake."[18]

Because being food insecure is related to income, household resources, and access to healthy foods, it is by definition related to poverty.[19] While one does not have to be poor to experience food insecurity, being food insecure is highly correlated with low income. The USDA reports the results of the U.S. Food Security Scale, which is part of the Census Bureau's Current Population Survey. The survey measures the level of food insecurity experienced by individuals and families, including children. Roughly 13% of the population—42 million people—are considered food insecure. A quarter of these households are considered to have very low food security. Food insecurity is highest among households with children headed by single mothers; black and Latino households also have a higher prevalence of food insecurity than white households. Furthermore, people living in nonmetropolitan areas are most likely to be food insecure.[20]

Food insecurity is related to both inadequate quantity and quality of food. When resources are limited, households may trade quality for quantity to avoid hunger. Nutrient-dense, energy-sparse foods (fruits, vegetables, and dairy) are generally more expensive than low-nutrient, energy-dense foods (refined grains, added sugars, and added saturated/trans fats). Therefore, food insecurity is not always connected to hunger. As pediatricians Debra Frank and John Cook note, "Although a young child subsisting on cheap 'junk food' may not cry from hunger, total intake of both macronutrients (calories and protein) and micronutrients may be insufficient for normal growth, leading to stunted growth (nutritional short stature) and underweight for age or height."[21]

The inability to afford healthy, nutrient-rich foods is also linked to obesity. While obesity rates have risen dramatically in the past 30 years among adults and children from all socioeconomic groups, it disproportionately affects people of lower socioeconomic and education levels and those from minority groups. In addition to the tradeoffs that low-income households make to reduce food costs (e.g., buying low-cost, high-calorie food rather than more expensive, healthier, lower-calorie foods to stretch food budgets), these households are also more likely than higher-income ones to live in *food deserts*, where healthier foods simply are not available. The USDA defines a food desert as "a part of the country vapid of fresh fruit, vegetables, and other healthful whole foods, usually found in impoverished areas. This is largely due to a lack of grocery stores, farmers' markets, and healthy food providers."[22] To qualify as a "low-access community," at least 500 people and/or at least 33% of the census tract's population must reside more than 1 mile from a supermarket or large grocery store (for rural census tracts, the distance is more than 10 miles).[23]

Particularly for young children, food insecurity can have a significant impact on development.[24] Comparisons of children under the age of three living in households with food insecurity with those in food-secure homes show that food-insecure children have worse overall health and more hospitalizations. Children and adolescents living in food-insecure homes are also more likely to be iron deficient, which can impact their energy and attention.[25] The stress associated with food insecurity can also have a significant effect on child health.

In adults, food insecurity is associated with chronic disease, such as diabetes and hypertension (high blood pressure). Food-insecure adults often report that they cannot afford balanced meals and often cut or skip meals. Replacement of fruits and vegetables with inexpensive carbohydrates raise glycemic (blood sugar) levels in adults predisposed to diabetes. Additionally, food insecurity is extremely stressful. Stress generally raises the body's level of cortisol, a hormone naturally released under stressful conditions; excessive cortisol can contribute to the development of diabetes and cardio-vascular disease.[26] Food insecurity among adults also affects health care utilization. One study found that the risk for admission to the hospital for hypoglycemia increased 27% in the last week of the month for a low-income population versus a high-income popu-lation. The study authors attribute this difference to food insecurity and the exhaustion by low-income households of food budgets by the end of the month.[27]

▶ Education

While perhaps not as obviously related to health as access to health care and food security, research continues to demonstrate that educational level is closely cor-related with health. Compared with college graduates, those who have not completed high school are more than four times as likely to be in fair or poor health. Children's health is also influenced by parental education: children of parents who have not finished high school are six times as likely to be in fair or poor health as children of college graduates.[28] Health economists have suggested that four additional years of educational attainment can reduce the risk of multiple health outcomes including mortality, heart disease, and diabetes, as well as self-reported poor health status and the number of sick days used.[29] The pathways by which education influences health are quite complex. They are thought to include differences between the more edu-cated and the less educated in health knowledge, literacy, and behavior; the role of educational attainment in employment opportunities and income; and education's effect on sense of control, social standing, and social support. **FIGURE 4.9** explains the multiple pathways from educational attainment to health.

At the same time, the pathways between education and health are not unidi-rectional. Health also influences educational attainment. As we discuss later in the chapter, childhood lead poisoning and asthma can significantly impede educational attainment. Children who suffer from chronic disease, disability, and mental health

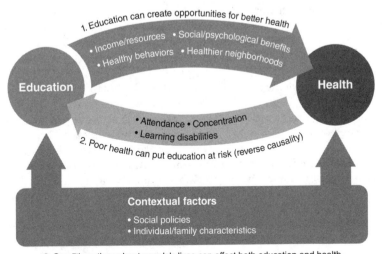

3. Conditions throughout people's lives can affect both education and health

FIGURE 4.9 How are education and health linked?

Reproduced from Center on Health and Society, Why education matters to health, April 2014. https://www.rwjf.org/en/library/research/2014/04/why-education-matters-to-health.html.

disorders are likely to experience disruptions in school functioning, limiting school achievement. Disadvantaged children who are poor, homeless, or who live in stressful and unstable home environments are also likely to suffer from increased absenteeism and interrupted learning.

Health disparities are closely associated with differences in educational opportunity and achievement. For example, health economist Janet Currie reviewed a range of common early childhood physical and mental health conditions known to affect cognitive skills and behavior and for which there are documented racial disparities (lead poisoning, asthma, anemia and iron deficiency, and attention-deficit hyperactivity disorder [ADHD]). She also studied maternal health conditions and behaviors (maternal depression and breastfeeding) believed to influence child cognitive and social functioning. Currie concludes that as much as a quarter of the school readiness gap between black and white children "might be attributable to health conditions or health behaviors of both mothers and children."[30] She suggests a range of policy responses that may help to reduce these health and educational disparities (including improving access to health care for low-income mothers and children; expansion of early childhood education and development programs that combine multiple services, such as health, child development, and parenting supports; family-based services such as home-visiting programs for high-risk families; and linking nutritional supports like the Special Supplemental Nutrition Program for Women, Infants and Children [WIC] to health care).[31] We further explore some of these programs and policies in other chapters.

▶ Employment

Like education, employment (and unemployment) are key factors in health through multiple mechanisms. Good jobs provide enough income to allow an individual or family to live in a healthy neighborhood, purchase nutritious food, and have access to quality health care. Additionally, since roughly half of Americans receive their health insurance through employment, a job serves as an important gateway to health care. Just as employment is protective of health, unemployment can harm it. The unemployed are 54% more likely to be in poor or fair health. They are also at high risk for stress-related conditions such as heart disease and stroke and to be diagnosed with depression.[32]

But even those who are employed may suffer the health consequences of low-paying, low-quality work. In 2014, 9.5 million people were classified as "working poor," meaning that they spent at least 27 weeks or more in a year in the labor force (working or looking for work), but their incomes nonetheless fell below the federal poverty level.[33] While the majority of the working poor have full-time jobs, they work in very low-wage jobs. Nearly one-third of American workers are in jobs in which the hourly rate is so low that, even working full time for the full year, their annual earnings would place them below the federal poverty level. Low-wage workers are disproportionately female, young, black, or Hispanic.[34]

In addition, many of the working poor cycle in and out of involuntary unemployment, as many low-wage jobs are unstable. Working in a low-wage job has four important consequences for health. First, low-wage workers are more likely to be exposed to dangerous and unhealthy working conditions. Notably, racial and ethnic minorities are more likely to work in jobs with higher risk of injury.[35] Second, many low-wage jobs do not provide workers with affordable health insurance. Third, due to inflexible work schedules and working conditions, access to health care may be impeded. Finally, workers in low-wage jobs are less likely to have access to paid sick and family leave. Indeed, the U.S. is the only country among 41 developed nations that has no nationwide requirement that employers provide some form of paid parental leave.[36] Because many low-wage jobs are part time and/or contingent, low-wage workers are least likely to work for employers that voluntarily provide paid leave. Because women are also more likely to work part time due to caretaking responsibilities, they are less likely than men to have access to health and leave benefits.[37]

▶ Safe and Affordable Housing

Those who work low-wage jobs also struggle with finding affordable, safe housing. Research continues to demonstrate the many ways in which access to safe, affordable housing is a major determinant of health. The unavailability of affordable housing affects health in at least two significant ways: (1) a high percentage of income devoted to rent may mean cutting back on other necessities, notably food and medical expenses; and (2) low-income tenants may accept substandard and unhealthy housing conditions when safe, affordable housing is unavailable. The lack of safe affordable housing in the U.S. is well documented. The National Low-Income Housing Coalition (NLIHC) estimates that the nation has a shortage of 7.4 million affordable rental homes for extremely low-income households (defined as "households with income at or below the poverty guideline or 30% of area median income, whichever is higher") and that there are only 35 affordable units for every 100 of these households. Housing is generally considered affordable if a family spends less than 30% of its income on rent or to purchase a home. Seventy-one percent of extremely low-income households spend more than half of their income on rent and utilities.[38] The number of renters increased 26% from 2006 to 2016, while homeownership decreased more than 5%. The wage required to afford a two-bedroom apartment in the U.S. is $21.21, nearly $14 higher than the federal minimum wage of $7.25 and $4.83 higher than the average hourly wage of $16.38 earned nationwide.[39]

Affordable Housing and Health

The gap between accessible affordable housing and the number of individuals and families needing it creates a range of health-related problems. First, it contributes to homelessness, which is highly correlated with poor health. The homeless have increased risk of infectious disease and chronic illness. Nearly half of homeless individuals have a chronic health problem. Rates of mental health and substance use disorders are also higher for the homeless, as is use of the emergency room as the primary source of health care. Homeless individuals also have a shortened lifespan.[40] Second, the affordable housing gap exacerbates the problem of eviction and housing instability. Housing instability has been shown to have particularly negative health effects for low-income mothers and children. In a study of the effects of eviction on families, researchers Matthew Desmond and Rachel Tolbert Kimbro found that:

> Compared to those not evicted, mothers who were evicted in the previous year experienced more material hardship, were more likely to suffer from depression, reported worse health for themselves and their children, and

reported more parenting stress. Some evidence suggests that at least two years after their eviction, mothers still experienced significantly higher rates of material hardship and depression than peers.[41]

Children who live in neighborhoods with unaffordable housing and who experience housing instability tend to have worse health and are more likely to have behavioral and school problems.[42]

Third, renters who are unable to pay their rent each month because of inadequate income and competing bills, such as for food or heat, are subject to the phenomenon known as "heat or eat." A family who pays a disproportionate percentage of household income for housing has less available income for other necessities. Low-income families with high housing and utility costs spend less on food, especially in the winter when utility costs are at their highest.[43] As discussed earlier, poor nutrition adversely affects health and development, especially for children. The heat or eat phenomenon is described in greater detail below.

Fourth and finally, the overall lack of affordable housing promotes health-harming housing conditions, including overcrowding (linked with greater risk of infectious disease and psychological distress), and acceptance of unsanitary and unsafe housing conditions over homelessness. In other words, an unhealthy and unsafe roof over one's head may be better than no roof at all. We detail some of these health-harming housing hazards below.

Health-Harming Housing Hazards

In addition to a shortage of affordable housing, the U.S. also suffers from a lack of available housing that has been built and maintained with health in mind, particularly in low-income neighborhoods. In a 2009 report, the U.S. Surgeon General defined a healthy home as "sited, designed, built, renovated, and maintained in ways that support the health of residents."[44] Yet a study by the U.S. Department of Housing and Urban Development showed that 23 million housing units have lead-based paint hazards, 17 million have high exposure to indoor allergens, and 6 million have moderate to severe infrastructure problems. The health burden from these housing problems include injury (especially for children and the elderly); respiratory illness such as asthma, chronic obstructive pulmonary disease, and emphysema from indoor exposure to pollutants; and childhood lead poisoning from exposure to lead in paint, water, and soil.[45]

As is likely unsurprising to you at this stage, these health burdens are not distributed equally across the population. Blacks are 1.7 times more likely as whites to live in homes with severe physical problems, and low-income people are 2.2 times more likely to live in substandard housing. Low-income households are also more likely to be poorly insulated, leading to the environment being too warm or too cool and to use of less safe forms of heating (e.g., space heaters).[46] Substandard housing conditions are shaped by social forces as well as local, state, and federal policies. For example, housing safety laws may be less likely to be enforced in low-income neighborhoods, leaving poor tenants with little recourse.[47] Specific health disparities associated with housing hazards have been well documented, particularly in low-income children. A few of these disparities are detailed in the following sections.

Lead Poisoning

While the overall burden of lead poisoning has diminished substantially in the past 20 years, racial- and socioeconomic-based lead-poisoning disparities have not.

Black children, low-income children, and children enrolled in Medicaid continue to have higher rates of lead poisoning than other children.[48] These disparities are driven by a number of factors. While the U.S. banned the use of lead in paint in 1978, homes built before 1978 are likely to have been painted with lead paint. If a home is in disrepair, the lead paint is more likely to chip and produce dust, which can then be ingested by children. Low-income children are more likely to live in older housing that is in disrepair.

Childhood lead poisoning is most often caused by exposure to dust and paint chips from interior surfaces of homes with deteriorating lead-based paint. Young children and babies are most at risk for lead poisoning because they crawl on the floor, exposing them to lead dust and paint chips. Because babies and toddlers engage in hand to mouth activities—exploring their world through putting things in their mouths—they are likely to ingest lead dust and chips more easily. In addition, because brain development is so rapid in the first six years of life, children's developing brains are more susceptible to the toxic effects of lead.

Overlaps between housing needs and food needs may also be at the root of the childhood lead-poisoning disparities. Deficiencies in both iron and calcium are thought to result in increased absorption of lead from the gut. Low-income children are more likely to experience food insecurity, and thus anemia and calcium deficiencies, which may increase their lead uptake.[49] Lead poisoning has serious, life-long consequences for health, development, cognition, and behavior. See **FIGURE 4.10**.

In addition to poisoning from lead paint, exposure to lead in water is also of concern. The water crisis in Flint, Michigan, which began in 2014, helped to raise awareness about the dangers of old pipes leaching lead into drinking water. In Flint, residents were exposed to high levels of lead in their drinking water after the town changed its water source—in order to save money—from Detroit's city water to the Flint River. Because the water was not properly treated, lead from pipes leading into

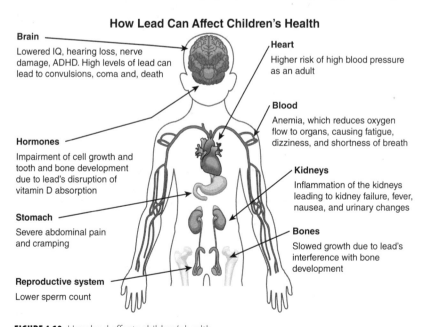

How Lead Can Affect Children's Health

Brain
Lowered IQ, hearing loss, nerve damage, ADHD. High levels of lead can lead to convulsions, coma and, death

Heart
Higher risk of high blood pressure as an adult

Blood
Anemia, which reduces oxygen flow to organs, causing fatigue, dizziness, and shortness of breath

Hormones
Impairment of cell growth and tooth and bone development due to lead's disruption of vitamin D absorption

Kidneys
Inflammation of the kidneys leading to kidney failure, fever, nausea, and urinary changes

Stomach
Severe abdominal pain and cramping

Bones
Slowed growth due to lead's interference with bone development

Reproductive system
Lower sperm count

FIGURE 4.10 How lead affects children's health.

Data from Calderone J, Gould S. Here's how lead is poisoning American children. *Business Insider.* March 7, 2016. http://www .businessinsider.com/lead-health-child-flint-michigan-body-pollution-water-2016-3.

homes from the street leached toxic levels of lead into the drinking water. Forty-one percent of residents in Flint live below the federal poverty level and 56% are black. After city, state, and federal government officials failed to recognize the problem and address it in a timely manner, many viewed their failure to act as systemic racism. In 2017, the Michigan Civil Rights Commission issued a report, "The Flint Water Crisis: Systemic Racism through the Lens of Flint," suggesting that "deeply embedded institutional, systemic and historical racism" contributed to governmental officials' decision to tap the Flint River as a cost-saving measure without due regard for the health consequences for Flint's population.[50] The Flint crisis has led to renewed calls for improving lead safety in homes and water, but few municipalities and states have the resources to undergo systematic remediation programs.

Housing Related Asthma Triggers

Another common housing-related health hazard is exposure to indoor pollutants that serve as "triggers" for asthma. Both the development of asthma and the severity of asthma are thought to be related to environmental triggers. Asthma is a chronic respiratory disease causing episodes of wheezing, coughing, and shortness of breath; if severe, it can be fatal. Asthma prevalence has doubled in the past two decades, and asthma accounts for over 10 million office visits, 400,000 hospitalizations, and 10 million missed days of work each year.[51] Asthma triggers include poor ventilation, dust mites, pet dander, cockroach and mice feces, and mold. Housing that has not been well maintained is especially prone to these triggers, and economically disadvantaged families who disproportionately live in substandard housing are at higher risk for asthma.

A study in New York City found that blacks and Hispanics were more likely to live in housing units with significant structural and maintenance problems, including water leaks that can lead to mold, chipping paint, broken plaster, holes in surfaces, and pest infestation—in other words, many of the types of substandard housing conditions that cause or exacerbate asthma.[52] Low-income families, particularly those in inner-city neighborhoods, are also at higher risk for exposure to outdoor pollutants such as transportation depots, industrial land use, and transfer stations, all of which can lead to or exacerbate asthma.[53]

Asthma is the most common chronic disease among children and 40% of asthma diagnosed in children is believed to be attributable to residential exposures.[54] Because these exposures are related to socioeconomic status, there are significant racial and socioeconomic disparities in rates of asthma. Surveillance data from the Centers for Disease Control and Prevention from 2001 to 2010 show that blacks and Puerto Ricans were significantly more likely than whites to have asthma. Blacks are three times more likely to visit the emergency department for asthma than whites.[55] **FIGURE 4.11** shows the multiple pathways between housing, environment, and asthma.

Asthma is also a leading medical cause of chronic school absenteeism. Asthma flare-ups may cause children to miss school to receive medical attention, including spending time in the emergency department or hospital for particularly severe episodes. Low-income children are more likely to have poorly controlled asthma, leading to flare ups. Poorly controlled asthma is also associated with problems with attention, cognition, and hyperactivity, which in turn can lead to poor academic performance.[56] Thus, asthma disparities not only contribute to poor health, they perpetuate inequalities in educational opportunity for disadvantaged children. Like childhood lead poisoning, which effects physical, cognitive, and behavioral

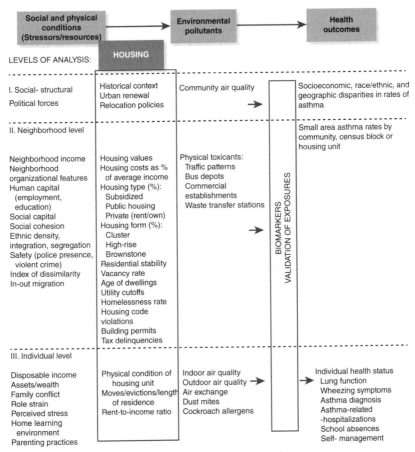

FIGURE 4.11 Links between environmental exposures and health outcomes mediated by housing.

Reproduced from Rauh VA, Landrigan PJ, Claudio L. Housing and health intersection of poverty and environmental exposures, *Annals of the N.Y. Academy of Sciences*. 2008;1136: 276–288.

functioning and thus can disrupt learning, asthma disparities exacerbate racial and socioeconomic inequality by reducing educational and economic opportunity for low-income children of color.

Energy Access

In addition to environmental exposures from substandard housing conditions, low-income families also experience an increased burden of utility shutoffs, in which their utilities, heat, water, and/or electricity are discontinued for some portion of the year. Lower-income households, who are more likely to live in older, less energy-efficient homes, spend on average 7.2% of their income on utility bills, while higher-income households spend roughly 2.3% of income on these bills.[57] Difficulty paying utility bills leaves lower-income households vulnerable to the phenomenon of "heat or eat" described earlier—the untenable of choice of paying the utility bill to keep the heat on in the winter, or putting food on the table. Exposure to very high or very low indoor temperatures can have significant effects on health. For example, exposure to cold temperatures is associated with increased risk of cardiovascular disease and asthma exacerbation.[58]

The "heat or eat" phenomenon has also been associated with "failure to thrive" in children. Failure to thrive broadly describes children who weigh less than the fifth percentile for their age, or who show a chronic pattern of poor weight gain. Failure to thrive in low-income children whose families are experiencing utility shutoff may occur because prolonged exposure to cold temperatures puts a child at risk for hypothermia, causing weight loss and neurological damage. Hypothermia increases metabolic rate and shivering to restore normal body temperature, which in turn results in more calorie burn-off. In other words, being cold increases calorie expenditure; this is particularly true for children. Thus, malnutrition is the end result of both food insecurity and utility insecurity.[59] Energy insecurity also places low-income families at risk for injury. Families may choose alternative heat sources for warmth, such as cooking stoves, wood-burning stoves, and space heaters, which are associated with greater risk for burns, fires, and respiratory illness.

▶ Neighborhoods

Like housing, neighborhoods play a key role in the health of individuals, families, and communities. The physical neighborhood, like a home, has implications for a range of health-related opportunities and disadvantages. These include such things as proximity to traffic, walkability, access to parks, availability of healthy food, and mixed-use development. It is not difficult to see that the structure of one's neighborhood can significantly affect health. Neighborhoods with sidewalks promote walking; mixed-use development promotes retail markets that are more like to offer healthy foods; parks improve air quality and provide exercise opportunities. Public health officials suggest that the built environment—the physical parts of where we live, work, and play, such as homes, buildings, streets, open spaces, and infrastructure—is crucial to improving population health. Neighborhood planning and design can make individual choices, such as eating healthier food and exercise, the easy choice rather than an uphill battle. Because low-income neighborhoods tend to experience more crime and violence, are often racially segregated with high concentrations of poverty, and lack many of the healthy attributes described above (sidewalks, parks, and access to healthy food), opportunities for health are severely curtailed. For example, fear of crime may drive parents in low-income neighborhoods to discourage their children from playing outdoors, and residents in neighborhoods without safe sidewalks are less likely to walk.

Racial and economic segregation are also associated with worse health outcomes. Studies show correlations between neighborhood disadvantage and cardiovascular disease, obesity, depression, cancer, and risk behaviors such as smoking, early sex, and substance abuse. Life expectancy can vary by as much as 25 years between neighborhoods, even ones just a handful of miles apart.[60] This association has led researchers to suggest that your health may be more a function of your zip code than your genetic code. **FIGURE 4.12** shows the differences in life expectancy in New Orleans, Louisiana, based on neighborhood or region of the city.

These health disparities are thought to be the result of greater exposure in segregated neighborhoods to poverty, violence, stress, indoor and outdoor environmental pollutants, and structural problems with the built environment. Historic racial segregation has left a legacy of multiple structural barriers for people living in

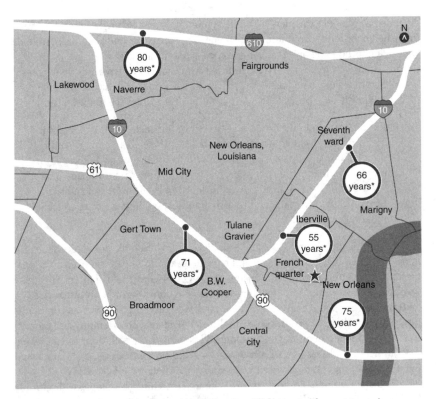

FIGURE 4.12 Map of New Orleans, Louisiana, showing differences in life expectancy by different regions of the city.

low-income neighborhoods, particularly for racial and ethnic minorities, including poor access to quality educational opportunities, employment, and health care. One study found that in metropolitan areas, 76% of black children and 69% of Latino children live in worse neighborhood conditions than the worst-off white children.[61]

Moving to a lower poverty neighborhood appears to improve well-being and life opportunities for low-income children. A 2015 study by Chetty, Hendren, and Katz found that children under the age of 13 whose low-income families were offered the opportunity to move to a lower poverty neighborhood, through the "Moving to Opportunity" experiment conducted by the U.S. Department of Housing and Urban Development, were more likely to go to a higher quality college and to have higher earnings in adulthood.[62] Because education and income are highly correlated with health outcomes, living in lower poverty neighborhoods that present opportunities for quality education and higher earnings also provide opportunities for better health.

▶ Environmental Justice and Climate Change

Just as homes and neighborhoods can create and reinforce disparate exposures that perpetuate health inequalities, pathogens caused by environmental toxins and the effects of climate change are not evenly distributed across populations. Research continues to demonstrate that "place matters" to health at multiple levels—from the home you live in to the neighborhood surrounding your home to the air, water, and land that surrounds your neighborhood. People of color and socioeconomically disadvantaged communities are more likely to be exposed to hazardous waste and other environmental toxins.[63] Spatial planning and zoning play a key role in the location of such hazards and the populations who will be exposed to them.[57] As one environmental health researcher notes:

> Vulnerable communities are used (directly or indirectly) to host social and environmental disamenities and externalities through planning, zoning, industrial siting, infrastructure and development inequities…There is an underdevelopment and/or destabilization in the growth, health, and quality of life of host communities overburdened by environmental and social externalities and spatially and socially bounded by limited access to environmental amenities.[64]

Economically disadvantaged communities and vulnerable populations are also more burdened by climate change and natural disasters. A 2017 report by National Oceanic and Atmospheric Administration (NOAA) confirmed that 2016 was the warmest year on record and that climate change is contributing to unusual weather patterns, storms, and sea level rise, which can have a disastrous impact on communities.[65] Climate change also affects health through heat-related morbidity and mortality due to rising temperatures and prolonged heat waves, air pollution, and increased risk of infectious disease, especially water- or vectorborne diseases, and trauma and mental health impacts of environmental disasters.[66] Refer to **FIGURE 4.13**.

Relatively vulnerable populations—the elderly, children, people with chronic health conditions, and those living in more marginalized communities—are most at risk for harm from climate change–related events. Hurricane Katrina, an extremely

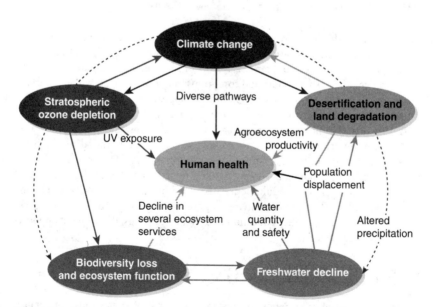

FIGURE 4.13 Climate change and health.

Reproduced from World Health Organization. Climate change and health. http://www.who.int/globalchange/climate/en/.

destructive storm that hit the Gulf Coast of the U.S. in 2005, exemplified the disproportionate toll that natural disasters can take on vulnerable populations. Of the roughly 1,400 Katrina-related deaths in Louisiana, fatalities were largest among the disabled, those living in nursing homes, and those from poor communities without the resources to relocate during the storm. One study reported that 49% of the fatalities were people age 75 or older and that the mortality rate among blacks was 1.7 to 4 times higher than among whites.[67]

The economic toll of the storm also disproportionately affected poor and vulnerable people, who were less likely to be able to rebuild their homes or who were dislocated from public housing that was never reopened after the storm. Post-Katrina studies of evacuees have shown that many suffer from resulting mental health problems such as depression and posttraumatic stress disorder (PTSD).[68] Disaster preparedness with a focus on protection of vulnerable communities during and after adverse weather events will be critically important in the future to avoid the severe consequences that resulted from Hurricane Katrina. Severe weather events in 2017, such as Hurricanes Harvey, Irma, Jose, and Maria, and the multiple earthquakes in Mexico, demonstrate that catastrophic storms and natural disasters are likely to continue to wreak havoc on communities for years to come.

▶ Personal Safety and Exposure to Violence

In addition to environmental health concerns, it is important to recognize the impact of human-to-human harm to health through violence. In this section we explore that exposure from two sources: community violence and family violence.

Neighborhood Violence

Research shows that protracted exposure to neighborhood violence is associated with intensified reactivity and heightened cortisol (stress hormone) levels in children. This biological response is thought to indicate a child's heightened vigilance to potential threats.[69] In addition to increased stress and vigilance, exposure to neighborhood violence affects the health of adults and children in a number of ways. First, unsafe neighborhoods appear to reduce physical activity because children and adults may forgo recreational activities in the neighborhood if they are concerned about safety. Second, individuals and families may lack social support, important to health and well-being, and become isolated if they are afraid to leave their homes. Third, people living in neighborhoods with high rates of violence are more likely to have mental health disorders and substance use disorders, and engage in risk-taking behaviors.

It is estimated that two-thirds of children are exposed to different types of community violence by the age of 18. Children living in economically disadvantaged communities are more likely to be exposed to violence.[70] A study of mothers of young children in Baltimore found that over the course of a year, 30% had witnessed a person being shot, more than half saw someone beaten or stabbed, 76% had witnessed someone being arrested, and the majority had been awakened by gunfire or police. The mothers who had witnessed violence had worse health outcomes on five measures than those who had not: self-reported health, smoking, exercise, amount of sleep, and sleep interruption. The study suggested that the mothers' exposure to neighborhood violence not only affected their own health, but also had detrimental effects on their ability to parent their young children.[71]

Violence in the Family

Just as exposure to neighborhood violence plays an important role in health, violence within families—including child maltreatment and intimate partner violence—is a significant determinant of health. Child maltreatment can be defined as "behavior towards [a child] . . . which (a) is outside the norms of conduct, and (b) entails a substantial risk of causing physical or emotional harm. Behaviors included will consist of actions and omissions, ones that are intentional and ones that are unintentional." Four types of maltreatment are generally recognized, including physical abuse, sexual abuse, neglect (including educational neglect, medical neglect, and other forms), and emotional maltreatment.[72]

Childhood exposure to physical, sexual, and emotional abuse and neglect can have severe consequences for child development, as well as for adult health outcomes. Exposure to physical and sexual abuse puts children at high risk of chronic health problems, posttraumatic stress disorder (PTSD), eating disorders, substance abuse, and suicidality.[73] In 2014, approximately 702,000 children were reported to have been maltreated. Children under the age of three are most at risk. Reported rates of neglect are significantly higher than those for physical and sexual abuse: in 2014, while 7.1 per 1,000 children were reported as neglected, 1.6 were reported as physically abused, and 0.8 were reported as sexually abused.[74]

Although child abuse and neglect occur in families from all socioeconomic groups, it is more prevalent in poor and extremely poor families. Roughly three times as many black, Hispanic, and American Indian/Alaska Native children live in poverty as do white and Asian American children. Black and Native American children are overrepresented in the child welfare system: while black children make up 13.8% of the population, they make up 24.3% of the children in foster care; white children make up 51.9% of the population and 43.4% of children in foster care; Native American children make up 0.9% of the population; and 1.8% of the children in foster care.[75] Researchers attribute this overrepresentation to:

- Disproportionate and disparate needs of children and families of color, particularly due to higher rates of poverty
- Racial bias and discrimination exhibited by individuals (e.g., caseworkers, reporters of abuse)
- Child welfare system factors (e.g., lack of resources for families of color, caseworker characteristics)
- Geographic context, such as the region, state, or neighborhood[76]

Understanding the role of poverty and lack of access to resources in child abuse and neglect, as well as disparate systemic responses to reports of child maltreatment, are important in identifying appropriate policy changes geared toward reducing racial, ethnic, and socioeconomic disparities. Given the significant health consequences for children associated with abuse and neglect, more upstream preventive measures are required.

Like child maltreatment, intimate partner violence (IPV)—also often referred to as domestic violence—is an important contributor to poor health in victims. IPV is defined as a pattern of purposeful coercive behaviors that may include inflicted physical injury, psychological abuse, sexual assault, progressive social isolation, stalking, deprivation, intimidation, or threats. These behaviors are perpetrated by someone who is, was, or wishes to be involved in an intimate or dating relationship with an adult or adolescent victim and aims to establish control over the other partner.[77]

It is estimated that a quarter of all women will experience IPV in their lifetime. Although men may also be victims, women are far more likely to experience IPV; it is the leading cause of nonfatal injury to women in the U.S. In addition to risk of physical injury, victims of IPV are at greater risk for mental health problems such as depression, anxiety, and PTSD, as well as for substance abuse and smoking. Because IPV is based on exerting power and control over the victim physically, emotionally, and sexually, through social and financial isolation, coercion, and threats, escaping the relationship is quite complex. In fact, victims are most at risk for death when they seek to leave the relationship.[78] **FIGURE 4.14** demonstrates the dynamics of power and control in IPV.

Poverty, homelessness, and undocumented immigrant status are critical risk factors for IPV because they create significant barriers for victims to leave an abusive relationship. Lack of financial resources and/or no alternative housing (other than the streets) create a strong deterrence to leaving. Undocumented immigrants may fear reporting abuse out of concern that it could lead to deportation.

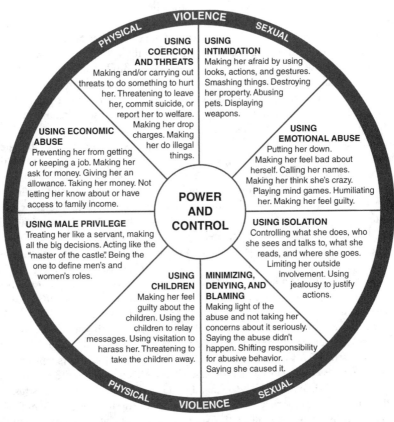

FIGURE 4.14 Power and control in physical and sexual violence.

Reproduced from Domestic Abuse Intervention Project. Power and control wheel of physical and sexual violence. Duluth, MN: Domestic Abuse and Intervention Project.

Children who are exposed to IPV in their homes also exhibit worse health and mental health outcomes. In young children these include failure to thrive, developmental delay, withdrawal, and sleep disruption. In older children, these include asthma, headaches, gastrointestinal issues, sleep disorders, aggressive behavior, and substance use. Exposure to IPV undermines a child's sense of safety and protection, leading him or her to see the world as dangerous and unpredictable and violence as a legitimate way to resolve conflict. This can have profound effects on a child's physical, mental, and emotional development and opportunities for a healthy life.

▶ Adverse Childhood Experiences and Toxic Stress

In 1998, Dr. Vincent Felitti and colleagues published a groundbreaking study on the relationship between health risk behavior and disease in adulthood and adverse childhood experiences (ACEs)—namely, exposure to childhood emotional, physical, or sexual abuse, household dysfunction (including exposure to intimate partner violence, parental substance abuse, and/or mental illness, and incarceration of a parent) and lack of basic necessities.[79] This study became known as the ACEs study and has been widely cited in recent years as further research has documented that ACEs not only drive poor adult health, they also appear to alter brain development in young children, leading to a host of negative outcomes.

The ACEs study found a "strong graded relationship between the breadth of exposure to abuse or household dysfunction during childhood and multiple risk factors for several of the leading causes of death in adults."[80] These include significantly heightened risk for substance abuse, depression, suicide, poor self-rated health, sexually transmitted disease, obesity, heart disease, cancer, chronic lung disease, liver disease, and skeletal fracture. More recently, researchers seeking to explain the pathways between ACEs and these negative adult health outcomes suggest that early childhood chronic stress, referred to as "toxic stress," actually creates "physiologic disruptions or biological memories that undermine the development of the body's stress response systems and affect the developing brain, cardiovascular system, immune system, and metabolic regulatory controls."[81] These "physiological disruptions" last into adulthood leading to lifelong disease and impairment.[82]

It is important to note that all stress is not bad stress. As noted earlier, stress produces the hormone cortisol, which, if properly regulated, helps us to focus on the task at hand. Our bodies are built around the idea of "fight or flight," or hyperarousal, to allow us to respond to a perceived threat or stressful situation. During times of acute stress, we go through a process known as allostasis, whereby our bodies make physiological adaptations to regulate and protect our bodies from exposure to stress. With toxic or chronic stress, our bodies are overloaded by the daily wear and tear of stress. This is known as "allostatic load." When this occurs, our physiological reactions to stress become progressively less effective in protecting our bodies from stress. When individuals feel that they do not have control over the stressors in their life, they are especially prone to allostatic load. Physician and epidemiologist Camara Phyllis Jones likens allostatic load to a car running at high RPMs continuously for weeks and months; eventually the car breaks down.[83]

Data from the 2016 National Survey of Children's health show that 46% of U.S. children under the age of 18 have had at least one ACE, while more than 20% have

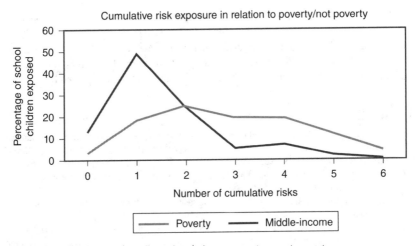

FIGURE 4.15 Cumulative risk exposure in relation to poverty or not poverty.

Data from Evans GW, English K. The environment of poverty: multiple stressor exposure. Psychophysiological stress, and socioemotional adjustment. *Child Development*. 2002;73(4):1238–1248.

had at least two.[84] Research also indicates that children who have had two or more ACES are significantly more likely to have a chronic health condition that requires special health care.[85] While adverse childhood experiences may occur at all socio-economic levels, children living in poverty who are exposed to multiple stressors—community crime and violence, food insecurity, overcrowding, unstable housing, lack of access to resources, environmental hazards, and underperforming schools—disproportionately suffer from toxic stress. **FIGURE 4.15** shows that cumulative risk exposure is higher for children living in poverty. Although the stress of poverty is most often associated with urban children, low-income rural children also experience toxic stress. A study of nine-year-old children showed that low-income children were much more likely to experience cumulative stress than middle-income nine-year-old children living in the same rural area.[86]

The daily wear and tear of these multiple stressors, or cumulative stress, can also affect daily functioning. Toxic stress affects what neuroscientists call executive functioning and self-regulation—the ability to plan ahead, focus, manage emotion, adapt to new situations, and resist impulses. These skills are critical for success in school, social relationships, and productivity. It should be noted that adults, like children, can experience toxic stress, and struggle with executive functioning as a result. Studies show that living in poverty with the constant worry of being unable to meet basic needs has a profound effect on adult cognitive functioning.[87]

▶ Conclusion

This chapter highlighted the multiple, and often overlapping, social and structural factors that influence health and that contribute to health disparities. You learned that the pathways between social and structural factors and health can be multifactorial as well as bidirectional. Poverty, which itself is a strong indicator for poor health, may include multiple subfactors—such as substandard housing, exposure to environmental hazards and violence, and poor access to health care and education—that also can lead to poor health. Poverty can also create a vicious cycle, reducing a person's opportunity for educational achievement—which is associated with poor health—while poor health also contributes to low educational achievement. In the next chapter, we investigate how effective existing safety net programs, laws, and policies are at addressing the social and structural barriers to health that were explored here.

References

1. Saez E, Zucman G. Wealth inequality in the United States since 1913: evidence from capitalized income tax data. *Quarterly Journal of Economics.* 2016;131(2):519–578. Available at: http://eml.berkeley.edu/~saez/SaezZucman2016QJE.pdf.
2. Dickman, SL, Himmelstein DU, Woolhandler, S. Inequality and the health-care system in the USA. *Lancet.* 2017;389:1431–1444.
3. Iceland, J. *Poverty in America: A Handbook.* Berkeley, CA: University of California Press; 2012: 20–28.
4. National Women's Law Center (NWLC). National snapshot: poverty among women & families, 2015. Washington, DC: NWLC. Available at: https://nwlc.org/resources/national-snapshot-poverty-among-women-families-2015/. Accessed September 26, 2017.
5. Centers for Disease Control and Prevention. Definitions: March 21, 2014. Available at: https://www.cdc.gov/nchhstp/socialdeterminants/definitions.html. Accessed September 26, 2017.
6. Health policy brief: the relative contribution of multiple determinants to health outcomes. *Health Affairs.* August 21, 2014. Available at: http://www.healthaffairs.org/healthpolicybriefs/brief.php?brief_id=123. Accessed September 26, 2017.
7. Berkman LF, Kawachi I, Glymour MM. *Social Epidemiology.* Oxford, U.K.: Oxford University Press; 2014: 2.
8. Bradley EH, Taylor LA. *American Health Care Paradox: Why Spending More is Getting Us Less.* New York, NY: Public Affairs; 2015; Bradley EH, Canavan M, Rogan E, et al. Variation in health outcomes: the role of spending on social services, public health, and health care, 2000–09. *Health Affairs.* 2016;35(5):760–768.
9. Collins SR, Gunja MZ, Beutel S. New U.S. census data show the number of uninsured Americans dropped by 4 million, with young adults making big gains. New York, NY: Commonwealth Fund; September 13, 2016. Available at: http://www.commonwealthfund.org/publications/blog/2016/sep/2015-census-data-insurance. Accessed October 9, 2017.
10. The Henry J. Kaiser Family Foundation. Key facts about the uninsured population (fact sheet); September 2017. Available at: http://files.kff.org/attachment/Fact-Sheet-Key-Facts-about-the-Uninsured-Population. Accessed October 9, 2017.
11. Griffith K, Evans L, Bor J. The Affordable Care Act reduced socioeconomic disparities in health care access. *Health Affairs.* 2017;36(8):1503–1510.
12. Griffith K, Evans L, Bor J. The Affordable Care Act reduced socioeconomic disparities in health care access. *Health Affairs.* 2017;36(8):1503–1510.
13. Griffith K, Evans L, Bor J. The Affordable Care Act reduced socioeconomic disparities in health care access. *Health Affairs.* 2017;36(8):1503–1510.
14. The Henry J. Kaiser Family Foundation. Data note: three findings about access to care. March 23, 2017. Available at: http://www.kff.org/medicaid/issue-brief/data-note-three-findings-about-access-to-care-and-health-outcomes-in-medicaid/. Accessed October 9, 2017.
15. Sommers BD, Long SK, Baicker, K. Changes in mortality after Massachusetts health care reform: a quasi-experimental study. *Annals of Internal Medicine.* 2014;160(9):585–593. Available at: http://annals.org/aim/article/1867050/changes-mortality-after-massachusetts-health-care-reform-quasi-experimental-study. Accessed October 9, 2017.
16. Hogan DR, Danaei G. Ezzati M, et al. Estimating the potential impact of insurance expansion on undiagnosed and uncontrolled chronic conditions. *Health Affairs.* September 2015;34(9):1554–1562.
17. U.S. Department of Agriculture (USDA), Economic Research Service. Definitions of food insecurity. Available at: https://www.ers.usda.gov/topics/food-nutrition-assistance/food-security-in-the-us/definitions-of-food-security/. Accessed October 9, 2017.

18. U.S. Department of Agriculture (USDA), Economic Research Service. Definitions of food insecurity. Available at: https://www.ers.usda.gov/topics/food-nutrition-assistance/food-security-in-the-us/definitions-of-food-security/. Accessed October 9, 2017.

19. Cook JT, Frank DA. Food security, poverty, and human development in the United States. *Annals of the New York Academy of Sciences.* 2008;1136:193–209, 195.

20. U.S. Department of Agriculture (USDA), Economic Research Service. Key statistics & graphics. Available at: https://www.ers.usda.gov/topics/food-nutrition-assistance/food-security-in-the-us/key-statistics-graphics.aspx. Accessed September 26, 2017.

21. U.S. Department of Agriculture (USDA), Economic Research Service. Key statistics & graphics. Available at: https://www.ers.usda.gov/topics/food-nutrition-assistance/food-security-in-the-us/key-statistics-graphics.aspx. Accessed September 26, 2017.

22. American Nutrition Association. USDA defines food deserts. *Nutrition Digest.* 2010;38(2). Available at: http://americannutritionassociation.org/newsletter/usda-defines-food-deserts. Accessed September 26, 2017.

23. American Nutrition Association. USDA defines food deserts. *Nutrition Digest.* 2010;38(2). Available at: http://americannutritionassociation.org/newsletter/usda-defines-food-deserts. Accessed September 26, 2017.

24. Rose-Jacobs R, Black MM, Casey PH, et al. Household food insecurity: associations with at-risk infant and toddler development. *Pediatrics.* 2008;121(1):65–72.

25. American Academy of Pediatrics, Council on Community Pediatrics, Nutrition Committee. Promoting food security for all children. *Pediatrics.* November 2015;136(5):1431–1438.

26. Seligman HK, Laraia BA, Kushel MB. Food insecurity is associated with chronic disease among low-income NHANES participants. *The Journal of Nutrition.* February 2010;140(2):304–310.

27. Seligman HK, Bolger AF, Guzman D, et al. Exhaustion of food budgets at month's end and hospital admissions for hypoglycemia. *Health Affairs.* January 2014;33(1):116–123.

28. Robert Wood Johnson Foundation Commission. Education and health. *Issue Brief 5*; April 2011. Available at: https://www.rwjf.org/content/dam/farm/reports/issue_briefs/2011/rwjf70447. Accessed October 9, 2017.

29. Cutler D, Lleras-Muney A. Education and health: evaluating theories and evidence. In: *Making Americans Healthier: Social and Economic Policy as Health Policy.* New York, NY: Russell Sage Foundation; 2008.

30. Currie J. Health disparities and gaps in school readiness. *Future of Children.* Spring 2005; 15(1):117–138.

31. Currie J. Health disparities and gaps in school readiness. *Future of Children.* Spring 2005; 15(1):117–138.

32. Robert Wood Johnson Foundation. How does employment—or unemployment—affect health? *Issue Brief*, March 2013. Available at: https://www.rwjf.org/content/dam/farm/reports/issue_briefs/2013/rwjf403360. Accessed September 26, 2017.

33. U.S. Bureau of Labor Statistics. A profile of the working poor; 2014. Available at: https://www.bls.gov/opub/reports/working-poor/2014/home.htm. Accessed September 26, 2017.

34. Levy BS, Wegman DH, Baron SL, et al. *Occupational and Environmental Health: Recognizing and Preventing Disease and Injury*, 6th ed. Oxford, U.K.: Oxford University Press; 2011: 70.

35. King TE, Wheeler MB, Bindman AB, eds. *Medical Management of Vulnerable and Underserved Patients: Principles, Practice, and Populations First Edition.* New York, NY: McGraw Hill; 2007: 213.

36. Pew Research Center. Among 41 nations, U.S. is the outlier when it comes to paid parental leave; September 26, 2016. Available at: http://www.pewresearch.org/fact-tank/2016/09/26/u-s-lacks-mandated-paid-parental-leave/. Accessed September 26, 2017.

37. The Henry J. Kaiser Family Foundation. Paid family leave and sick days in the U.S.: findings from the 2016 Kaiser/HRET employer health benefits survey; May 31, 2017. Available at: http://www.kff.org/womens-health-policy/issue-brief/paid-family-leave-and-sick-days-in-the-u-s-findings-from-the-2016-kaiser-hret-employer-health-benefits-survey/. Accessed September 26, 2017.

38. National Low Income Housing Coalition (NLIHC). The gap: a shortage of affordable homes; March 2017. Available at: http://nlihc.org/sites/default/files/Gap-Report_2017_interactive.pdf. Accessed October 9, 2017.

39. National Low-Income Housing Coalition (NLIHC). Out of reach 2017: how much do you need to earn to afford a modest apartment in your state? Available at: http://nlihc.org/oor. Accessed October 9, 2017.

40. Schanzer B, Dominguez B, Shrout P, Caton CLM. Homelessness, health status, and health care use. *American Journal of Public Health*. March 2007;97(3):464–469.

41. Desmond M, Tobert Kimbro R. Eviction's fallout: housing, hardship, and health. *Social Forces*. September 2015;94(1):295–324, 297.

42. Robert Wood Johnson Foundation. Where we live matters for our health: the links between housing and health. *Issue Brief 2: Housing and Health*; September 2008: 6.

43. Frank, DA, Neault NA, Skalicky A, et al. Heat or eat: the low income energy assistance program and nutritional and health risks amongst children less than three years of age. *Pediatrics*. 2006;118(5):1293–1302.

44. U.S. Department of Health and Human Services. Call to action to promote healthy homes. Washington, DC: Office of the Surgeon General; June 2009: i.

45. President's Task Force on Environmental Health Risks and Safety Risks to Children, Healthy Homes Workgroup. Advancing healthy housing: a strategy for action; 2013: 13–14.

46. Krieger J, Higgins DL. Housing and health: time again for public health action. *American Journal of Public Health*. May 2002;92(5):758–768, 760.

47. Tobin Tyler E. When are laws strictly enforced? Criminal justice, housing quality, and public health. *Health Affairs Blog*. November 5, 2015. Available at: http://healthaffairs.org/blog/2015/11/05/when-are-laws-strictly-enforced-criminal-justice-housing-quality-and-public-health/. Accessed October 9, 2017.

48. American Academy of Pediatrics Policy Statement. Lead exposure in children: prevention, detection, and management. *Pediatrics*. October 2005;116(4):1036–1046, 1037.

49. Tobin Tyler E, Conroy KN, Fu C, Sandel M. Housing: the intersection of affordability, safety and health. In: Tobin Tyler E, Lawton E, Conroy C, Sandel M, et al., eds. *Poverty, Health and Law: Readings and Cases for Medical-Legal Partnership*. Durham, NC: Carolina Academic Press; 2012: 242.

50. The Michigan Civil Rights Commission. The Flint water crisis: systemic racism through the lens of Flint; February 17, 2017. Available at: http://www.michigan.gov/documents/mdcr/VFlintCrisisRep-F-Edited3-13-17_554317_7.pdf. Accessed October 9, 2017.

51. Newacheck PW, Halfon N. Prevalence, impact, and trends in childhood disability due to asthma. *Archives of Pediatric and Adolescent Medicine*. 2000;154:287–293.

52. Rosenbaum E. Racial/ethnic differences in asthma prevalence: the role of housing and neighborhood environment. *Journal of Health and Social Behavior*. June 2008;49(2):131–145, 132.

53. Rosenbaum E. Racial/ethnic differences in asthma prevalence: the role of housing and neighborhood environment. *Journal of Health and Social Behavior*. June 2008;49(2):131–145, 132.

54. Robert Wood Johnson Foundation. Where we live matters for our health: the links between housing and health. *Issue Brief 2: Housing And Health*. September 2008: 6.

55. Centers for Disease Control and Prevention, National Surveillance of Asthma: United States, 2001–2010. Available at: https://www.cdc.gov/nchs/data/series/sr_03/sr03_035.pdf.

56. Basch CE. Healthier students are better learners: a missing link in school reforms to close the achievement gap. A Research Initiative of the Campaign for Educational Equity Teachers College, Columbia University. March 2010.

57. Energy Efficiency for All. Lifting the high energy burden in America's largest cities: how energy efficiency can improve low income and underserved communities; April 2016. Available at: http://energyefficiencyforall.org/sites/default/files/Lifting%20the%20High%20Energy%20Burden_0.pdf. Accessed October 9, 2017.

58. Energy Efficiency for All. Lifting the high energy burden in America's largest cities: how energy efficiency can improve low income and underserved communities; April 2016. Available at: http://energyefficiencyforall.org/sites/default/files/Lifting%20the%20High%20Energy%20Burden_0.pdf. Accessed October 9, 2017.

59. Frank, DA, Neault NA, Skalicky A, et al. Heat or eat: the low income energy assistance program and nutritional and health risks amongst children less than three years of age. *Pediatrics*. 2006;118(5):1293–1302.

60. Jutte DP, Miller JL, Erickson DJ. Neighborhood adversity, child health, and the role for community development. *Pediatrics.* March 2015;135(2):S48–S57.

61. Williams DR, Jackson PB. Social sources of racial disparities in health. *Health Affairs.* March/April 2005;24(2):325–334.

62. Chetty R, Hendren N, Katz LF. The effects of exposure to better neighborhoods on children: new evidence from the moving to opportunity experiment. Harvard University and National Bureau of Economic Research; May 2015.

63. Wilson SM. An ecologic framework to study and address environmental justice and community health issues. *Environmental Justice.* 2009;2(1):15–23, 15–16.

64. Maantay J. Zoning, equity, and public health. *American Journal of Public Health.* July 2001;91:1033–1041.

65. National Oceanic and Atmospheric Administration (NOAA). International report confirms 2016 was warmest year on record for the globe. Available at: http://www.noaa.gov/news/international-report-confirms-2016-was-warmest-year-on-record-for-globe. Accessed October 9, 2017.

66. Levy BS, Patz JA. *Climate Change and Health.* Oxford, U.K.: Oxford University Press; 2015.

67. Brunkard JN, Amulanda G, Ratard R. Hurricane Katrina deaths, Louisiana, 2005. *Disaster Medicine and Public Health Preparedness.* December 2008;2(4):215–223.

68. King RV, Polatin PB, Hogan D, Downs D, North CS. Needs assessment of Hurricane Katrina evacuees residing temporarily in Dallas. *Community Mental Health Journal.* 2016;52:18.

69. Theall KP, Shirtcliff EA, Dismukes AR, Wallace M, Drury SS. Association between neighborhood violence and biological stress in children. *JAMA Pediatrics.* 2017;171(1):53–60.

70. Aizer A. Neighbohood violence and urban youth. National Bureau of Economic Research; February 2008.

71. Johnson SL, Solomon BS, Shields WC, McDonald EM, McKenzie LB, Gielen AC. Neighborhood violence and its association with mothers' health: assessing the relative importance of perceived safety and exposure to violence. *Journal of Urban Health.* July 2009;86(4):538–550.

72. Child Trends. Databank Indicator: Child maltreatment. Available at: https://www.childtrends.org/indicators/child-maltreatment/. Accessed October 9, 2017.

73. The U.S. Department of Justice. Children exposed to violence; 2012. Available at: https://www.justice.gov/sites/default/files/defendingchildhood/cev-rpt-full.pdf.

74. The U.S. Department of Justice. Children exposed to violence; 2012. Available at: https://www.justice.gov/sites/default/files/defendingchildhood/cev-rpt-full.pdf.

75. Children's Bureau, Child Welfare Information Gateway. Racial disproportionality and disparity in child welfare. *Issue Brief;* October 2106. Available at: https://www.childwelfare.gov/pubPDFs/racial_disproportionality.pdf.

76. Children's Bureau, Child Welfare Information Gateway. Racial disproportionality and disparity in child welfare. *Issue Brief;* October 2106. Available at: https://www.childwelfare.gov/pubPDFs/racial_disproportionality.pdf.

77. Groves BM, Augustyn M, Lee D, Sawires P. *Identifying and Responding to Domestic Violence: Consensus Recommendations for Child and Adolescent Health.* San Francisco, CA: Family Violence Prevention Fund; 2002.

78. McAlister Groves B, Pilnik L, Tobin Tyler E, et al. Personal safety: addressing interpersonal and family violence in the health and legal systems. In: Tobin Tyler E, Lawton E, Conroy C, Sandel M, et al., eds. *Poverty, Health and Law: Readings and Cases for Medical-Legal Partnership.* Durham, NC: Carolina Academic Press; 2012.

79. Felitti VJ, Anda RF, Nordenberg D, et al. Relationship of childhood abuse and household dysfunction to many of the leading causes of death in adults: The Adverse Childhood Experiences (ACE) Study. *American Journal of Preventive Medicine.* 1998;14(4):245–258.

80. Felitti VJ, Anda RF, Nordenberg D, et al. Relationship of childhood abuse and household dysfunction to many of the leading causes of death in adults: The Adverse Childhood Experiences (ACE) Study. *American Journal of Preventive Medicine.* 1998;14(4):245–258.

81. Shonkoff JP, Garner AS, Committee on Psychosocial Aspects of Child and Family Health, Committee on Early Childhood, Adoption, and Dependent Care; Section on Developmental

and Behavioral Pediatrics. The lifelong effects of early childhood adversity and toxic stress. *Pediatrics*. 2012;129(1):232–243.

82. Shonkoff JP, Garner AS, Committee on Psychosocial Aspects of Child and Family Health, Committee on Early Childhood, Adoption, and Dependent Care; Section on Developmental and Behavioral Pediatrics. The lifelong effects of early childhood adversity and toxic stress. *Pediatrics*. 2012;129(1):232–243.

83. Goldberg D, Baxley EG, Fancher TL. Socioecologic determinants of health. *Health Systems Science*. AMA Education Consortium. 2017; 134–152, 140 (citing Camara Phyllis Jones).

84. Data Resource Center for Child and Adolescent Health. Indicator 6.13: How many children experienced one or more adverse childhood experiences from the list of 9 ACEs? Available at: http://childhealthdata.org/browse/survey/results?q=4783&r=1. Accessed December 6, 2017.

85. Centers for Disease Control and Prevention. Adverse childhood experiences. Available at: https://www.cdc.gov/violenceprevention/acestudy/index.html. Accessed December 6, 2017.

86. Evans GW, Brooks-Gunn J, Klebanov PK. Stressing out the poor: chronic physiological stress and the income-achievement gap. *Community Investments*. Fall 2011;23(2):22–27, 25.

87. Mani A, Mullainathan S, Shafir E, Zhao J. Poverty impedes cognitive function. *Science*. 2013;341:976–980.

PART III

Striving for Health Justice

Part III of this book includes three chapters focusing on existing programs and laws that help to promote health, system innovations and policy efforts intended to improve population health and reduce disparities, and advocacy strategies for advancing health justice at the systems level. Chapter 5 describes existing safety net programs and some health-related legal protections in the United States. Chapter 6 explores types of coordinated care systems that are needed to care for socially complex patients and populations, and Chapter 7 offers ways in which readers of this text can advocate for health justice.

Safety Net Programs and Legal Protections That Support Health

LEARNING OBJECTIVES

By the end of this chapter you will be able to:

- Describe general eligibility and program requirements for various government safety net programs, including those that provide access to income, health care, and food assistance.
- Analyze the role and adequacy of safety net programs in promoting population health and reducing health disparities.
- Discuss some of the legal protections that address the social determinants of health and describe the gaps in these protections.

▶ Introduction

So far, we have described the multiple social and structural forces, and also some broad legal doctrines, that affect health and contribute to health inequality. This chapter turns to existing government programs and systems that are designed to provide a safety net for vulnerable populations. These safety net programs include income supports, publicly funded health insurance and medical care, food and housing assistance, and more. In addition to the government safety net, this chapter also covers some select legal protections intended to protect health, safety, and well-being. While there are many laws that could be viewed as intended to promote health, we focus here on those that address specific social and structural barriers to health and safety as described in the chapter on social and structural barriers to health. These include protecting individuals who are wrongfully denied access to government benefits, those whose employment rights or right to safe housing have been violated, and justice system responses to family violence. As you read about the social safety net and these legal protections, ask yourself: how effective are these current programs and systems in protecting and promoting the health of vulnerable populations?

▶ The Structure of the Social Safety Net

Before describing specific safety net programs and legal protections, we start by explaining what we mean by the "safety net," who is eligible for safety net programs, who actually participates in it, and how effective it is in reducing poverty (or at least in ameliorating its effects).

What Is the Safety Net?

The term *safety net* is used to describe the combination of government programs that are designed to prevent individuals and families from falling into poverty. These programs include income supports such as welfare, tax credits, and unemployment insurance, as well as subsidies for food and housing, and publicly funded health insurance for eligible individuals.

Who Is Eligible for Safety Net Programs?

Safety net programs may have *categorical eligibility* requirements, *income eligibility* requirements, or both. Categorical eligibility means that a particular category of person is eligible—such as, children, people over age 65, or those with disabilities. In the United States, categorical eligibility has historically been determined by making a distinction between the "deserving" and "undeserving" poor. Many safety net programs have been constructed to assist those viewed as particularly vulnerable or deserving of government assistance: single mothers, children, the elderly, and the disabled. Able-bodied adults, regardless of income, have typically been regarded as undeserving of government assistance. Categories of people deemed deserving have evolved over time, and still remain controversial. For example, as discussed below in more detail, changes were made to the safety net in 1996 based on the idea that poor single mothers should be considered able-bodied adults, only deserving of government assistance if they demonstrated that they were working or engaged in education and job training.

Generally, income eligibility requirements are based on the *federal poverty guidelines*. Issued each year by the U.S. Department of Health and Human Services (DHHS), these guidelines are based on the *federal poverty threshold*, which is used to calculate the amount of income needed by an individual or family to meet a basic standard of living. **TABLE 5.1** shows the poverty guidelines for 2017. Safety net program eligibility is often based on a percentage of the federal poverty guideline. For example, eligibility for the Medicaid program may be based on a person's income being 138% (or less) of the federal poverty guideline. The federal poverty threshold is criticized as underestimating the number of people who live in poverty because its calculation of the cost of meeting basic needs is too low and does not account for a range of factors affecting actual standard of living, including geographic differences, dramatically different housing costs by region, and other expenses borne by individuals and families in the current economy.[1]

TABLE 5.1 2017 Poverty Guidelines for the 48 Contiguous States and the District of Columbia

Persons in Family/Household	Poverty Guideline
1	$12,060
2	$16,240
3	$20,420
4	$24,600
5	$28,780
6	$32,960
7	$37,140
8	$41,320

Federal Register, Annual Update of the HHS Poverty Guidelines. https://www.federalregister.gov/documents/2017/01/31/2017-02076/annual-update-of-the-hhs-poverty-guidelines.

What Is an Entitlement?

The media and policymakers often talk about the rising costs of entitlement programs, but what exactly is an entitlement and how is it different from other government benefits? Some safety net programs are structured to provide benefits to eligible people on a first-come, first-serve basis. The government appropriates a fixed amount of funding to support the benefit program, and when that funding is spent, there is no additional funding to support more benefits, even if all eligible individuals have not received the benefit. This is true, for example, for housing subsidies, as is described below. Other government benefits, however, are legal entitlements, meaning that by law, the government must supply the benefit to all eligible individuals, regardless of cost. There is, therefore, no cap on spending for the program; it is an open appropriation. As discussed below, Medicaid and Medicare are examples of entitlement programs.

Who Participates in Safety Net Programs?

The U.S. Census reports that in 2012, just over 52 million people, or about one-fifth of the population, participated in a major means-tested (i.e., income-based) government assistance program. Those without a high school diploma were most likely to participate (37.3%) compared with high school graduates (21.5%) and those with one or more years of college (9.6%). Just over 39% of participants were children. Average monthly participation rates were highest among blacks and Hispanics and

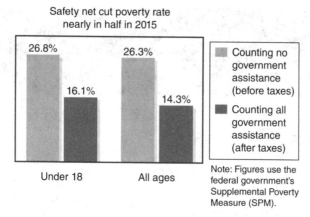

FIGURE 5.1 Safety net cut poverty rate nearly in half in 2015.

Data from Center for Budget and Policy Priorities. Safety net cut poverty nearly in half last year. September 14, 2016. https://www.cbpp .org/blog/safety-net-cut-poverty-nearly-in-half-last-year.

for single female-headed households with children (50%).[2] Immigrants may or may not have access to safety net programs depending on their legal status. Generally, undocumented immigrants are not eligible for safety net programs. For some safety net programs, such as TANF (welfare), Medicaid, and SNAP (food stamps), lawful permanent residents may apply only after waiting for five years.

Do Safety Net Programs Reduce Poverty?

While the average monthly benefit from safety net programs is quite modest, these programs have been shown to reduce poverty. The Census Bureau reports that the median monthly benefit across all programs was $404.[3] Yet, far more people would live below the federal poverty level if they did not have access to safety net programs. When counting government assistance provided through these programs as additional income, the poverty rate would be twice as high without the safety net. See **FIGURE 5.1**.

▶ Income Supports

In the chapters on health disparities and social and structural barriers to health, we described the strong correlation between income, poverty, and health. Higher income, particularly when it raises a person or family out of poverty, is a strong predictor of improved health outcomes. There are a number safety net programs designed to raise household income in order to prevent an individual or family from falling below the poverty line. Income supports are distributed across four main types of government programs: (1) The Temporary Assistance for Needy Families Program (TANF), a welfare program for very poor parents and children; (2) the Social Security Disability Insurance (SSDI) and Social Security Insurance (SSI) programs, which replace wage loss for individuals too disabled to work; (3) the Unemployment Insurance (UI) program, which provides partial wage replacement during temporary unemployment; and (4) the earned income tax credit (EITC), which serves to boost the income of low-wage workers by providing a tax refund for workers earning below a certain annual income.

The Temporary Assistance for Needy Families Program

The Temporary Assistance for Needy Families Program (TANF) program was created in 1996 as part of the Personal Responsibility and Work Opportunity Reconciliation Act (PRWORA). TANF replaced the Aid to Families with Dependent Children (AFDC) program, which was established in 1935 to provide cash welfare to poor single mothers and their children during the Great Depression. The new program was explicitly designed to "end welfare as we know it" by President William Clinton and by the U.S. Congress, based on concerns that the AFDC program was creating a "culture of dependency" on the government by its recipients. TANF is a federal program that provides block grants—essentially, a predetermined amount of money—to states to design their own welfare programs; states must contribute "maintenance of effort" dollars to support their programs. TANF shifted the focus of welfare away from cash assistance to needy families toward the use of government funding to support work and personal independence. The goals stated in the TANF statute are to: "(1) provide assistance to needy families so that children may be cared for in their own homes or in the homes of relatives; (2) end the dependence of needy parents on government benefits by promoting job preparation, work, and marriage; (3) prevent and reduce the incidence of out of wedlock pregnancies and establish annual numerical goals for preventing and reducing the incidence of these pregnancies; and (4) encourage the formation and maintenance of two parent families."[4]

To meet these goals, the law provides strict work requirements for recipients as well as time limits (a five-year lifetime limit on receipt of benefits). Studies of the TANF program show that the number of poor families receiving assistance has dropped dramatically over time as states have continued to reduce benefits. In 1996, 68 out of 100 poor families received TANF benefits; in 2015, 23 out of 100 poor families received TANF. During the "Great Recession" beginning in 2008, federal block grants did not increase as need increased. Some states responded to rising caseloads by cutting benefits and tightening restrictions. With an average monthly state TANF benefit of about $432 in 2016, purchasing power has dropped since 1996 as many states have failed to raise benefits to adjust for inflation.[5] Researchers have also found that the number of children living in extreme poverty (defined by The World Bank as households living on $2 or less per person per day[6]) doubled in the U.S. from 1.4 to 2.8 million between 1996 and 2011, indicating that lack of access to welfare assistance or inadequate benefits has led to severe deprivation for the most vulnerable families.[7]

Some states use federal TANF block grant funds to pay for subsidized child care for low-income working parents. States are permitted under federal law to use TANF funds directly for child care assistance or to transfer up to 30% of their TANF funds to the state's Child Care and Development Block Grant (CCDBG), another federal grant program to states. This assistance is a critically important factor in enabling parents—particularly women—to work, and it helps protect families from falling into poverty by reducing out-of-pocket expenses for child care, which can absorb a large portion of monthly income. For example, in 2016, one week of care for a single child at a child care center in the U.S. averaged $196 ($784 per month). Due to these high costs, one-fifth of all families spend more than a quarter of their income on child care.[8] In Massachusetts, where the annual cost of full-time child care for an infant in a child care center is $15,000, all of a minimum wage worker's earnings would be consumed by child care costs.[9]

After passage of PRWORA in 1996, many states expanded their child care assistance programs to support low-income parents as they transitioned into work. But funding for child care assistance has declined significantly in the past decade. From 2000 to 2015, TANF funds used by states for child care declined from $4 billion to $2.6 billion, with 19 states spending less than 10% of TANF funds on child care.[10] The National Women's Law Center reports that "in 2014, 1.4 million children were served by CCDBG in an average month, which was the lowest number since 1998, and 364,000 fewer children than in 2006."[11]

Without financial assistance, many low-income parents are forced to accept poorer quality child care in order to work. Studies show that low-income mothers are more likely to rely on informal, lower-quality care arrangements. However, when provided financial assistance, they are more likely to select child care centers that provide better opportunities for early learning.[12] Early child development and education programs have been shown to be particularly important to promote school readiness for low-income children, who often present at school as educationally behind their more affluent peers.[13] In addition, according to one study, children who participate in well-designed, responsive preschools have fewer behavioral problems in middle school.[14] As you have read earlier, educational success is highly correlated with good health outcomes and vice versa. Not only does access to quality child care enable parents to work and lead to a reduction in their stress, it supports critical early development and learning opportunities for their children, affecting kids' health and life course.

Social Security Disability Insurance and Social Security Insurance

As described in the chapter on health disparities, having a disability is closely associated with social context. Black and Hispanic adults are more likely to have a disability than are whites; those with lower educational levels and incomes are also more likely to be disabled. One in three blacks and one in four women were reported to have a disability; half of those living in a household with income below $15,000 report a disability.[15]

The Social Security Administration (SSA) administers the Social Security Disability Insurance (SSDI) and Social Security Insurance (SSI) programs, which provide wage replacement programs for individuals who are too disabled to work. Eligibility for the programs is based on federal disability criteria established by the SSA. SSDI provides benefits to disabled or blind individuals who are "insured" by workers' contributions to the Social Security trust fund, meaning that the claimant or a qualified family member must have worked a specified number of quarters with payment into the trust fund through payroll or self-employment taxes. SSI, on the other hand, provides benefits to disabled, blind, or aged (65 years or older) individuals with limited income and resources. There is no prior work history requirement. To qualify for disability insurance an individual must demonstrate that he or she is unable to engage in any "substantial gainful activity" by reason of any medically determinable physical or mental impairment or combination of impairments that has lasted or can be expected to last for a continuous period of not less than 12 months or to result in death. Children under age 18 may also be eligible for disability insurance to provide financial assistance to their families in caring for them. For children, instead of evaluating the ability to work or substantial gainful activity, SSA evaluates whether the child's impairments cause "marked and severe functional limitations."[16]

Economist David Autor points to flaws in the design of the SSDI program in particular, which he argues have led to unsustainable growth in the program. He argues that the program is ineffective in incentivizing less severely disabled workers to return to appropriate work, while at the same time failing to reserve longer-term benefits for the more severely disabled.[17] Another concern with the SSDI and SSI programs is that administrative barriers can cause significant hardship for poor disabled adults. Benefit applicants encounter long delays in the processing of their claims, with many claims being denied at initial determination by SSA, requiring the applicant to appeal. Long delays can be a significant hardship for disabled individuals who have no other source of income.[18]

Unemployment Insurance

The chapter on social and structural barriers to health outlined the role that employment plays in health and the detrimental effects of unemployment on health. The Unemployment Insurance (UI) program is designed to provide a financial buffer to those who have lost their jobs as they search for employment. It is administered jointly by the U.S. Department of Labor and the states to provide temporary, partial income replacement for workers who have lost their jobs through no fault of their own. States set eligibility and benefit levels. To qualify, a worker must certify that he or she is able to and is actively seeking work. UI benefits typically amount to about half of a worker's prior wages, up to a maximum benefit amount, and can be taken for a period up to 26 weeks. During the Great Recession, when the unemployment rate soared, most states extended the period for up to 99 weeks. While some policymakers were concerned that this extension would lead individuals to stop looking for work, some economists suggest that the extension did not affect job growth.[19]

The Earned Income Tax Credit

The earned income tax credit (EITC) is a federal tax credit for low- and moderate-income working people—those with children and earning below about $39,300 to $53,500 (depending on marital status and the number of children), and single adults without children earning below about $14,900. The EITC has two core goals: (1) encourage and reward work, and (2) reduce poverty. A worker's EITC grows with each additional dollar of wages until it reaches the maximum value. The EITC is refundable, meaning that if it exceeds a low-wage worker's income tax liability, the IRS will refund the balance. The average EITC for a family with children for tax year 2015 was $3,186. The Center for Budget Policy and Priorities—a nonpartisan research and policy institute in Washington, DC—estimates that in 2015, the EITC lifted 6.5 million people out of poverty and reduced the severity of poverty for another 21 million people.[20] Given the rise in income inequality in the past 35 years and its role in health inequality, income support programs, like those described here, may be critical in improving reducing health disparities.

▶ Health Care Programs

Medicaid

Unlike most other developed countries, the U.S. has not embraced a universal, government-funded health care safety net. Instead, it provides access to health insurance to some low-income individuals through the Medicaid program. Created in 1965 as part of President Lyndon Johnson's War on Poverty, the program was intended to provide a safety net for the very poor and disabled who otherwise could not afford health insurance or who lacked access to health care. Using both categorical and income eligibility criteria, the program covered low-income pregnant women, children, the disabled, and the elderly poor. In 2010, when the Affordable Care Act expanded federal eligibility for Medicaid, all individuals with an income below 138% of the federal poverty level—regardless of category (e.g., disability, age)—became eligible and states were required to cover them. But in a major case in 2012 (*National Federation of Independent Business v. Sebelius*), which challenged the Congress's power to require Medicaid expansion in all states, the U.S. Supreme Court held that Congress could not "coerce" states into expanding their Medicaid programs by threatening the loss of other federal Medicaid funding.[21] Given the choice to expand their Medicaid programs to single poor adults with generous support from the federal government, 32 states and the District of Columbia have expanded their programs, while 18 states have not (as of November 2017).[22]

Medicaid has always been structured as a joint federal-state program in which the federal government matches state funds on an open-ended basis. Apart from core federal standards for coverage and eligibility, states have great flexibility in designing and administering their Medicaid programs. Because Medicaid is an entitlement program, all individuals who are deemed eligible under federal and state requirements are guaranteed coverage. Medicaid now covers more than 70 million people, or one in five Americans. It is also the major source of coverage for long-term care for older Americans. In addition to providing insurance coverage to individuals, Medicaid finances a large segment of the health care system, including hospitals, nursing homes, community health centers, and physicians and other health care providers.[23]

As the Medicaid program's costs to the federal government and to state budgets have increased over time, some states have limited eligibility and coverage to the minimum federal requirements. As recently as the summer of 2017, Republicans have proposed changing Medicaid from a federal entitlement to a block granted program, similar to TANF, as well as significant cuts to funding to the states. Additionally, some states have proposed work requirements for receipt of Medicaid coverage, though these have not yet taken affect as of the time of this writing. As you can see, the question of who is deserving of government assistance, whether through income supports or through health insurance coverage, and how much assistance should be provided, are issues that remain hotly debated in the U.S.

Medicare

Like Medicaid, Medicare was created in 1965 to prevent a vulnerable group—older Americans—from going without health care. Unlike Medicaid, Medicare has no income eligibility requirements, but instead is based solely on whether or not an individual is categorically eligible. Also unlike Medicaid, Medicare has not been subjected to the frequent calls for reform, which most often involve reducing eligibility and funding cuts. Medicare beneficiaries—older Americans—are substantially stronger politically than Medicaid beneficiaries—the poor and disabled. Most individuals ages 65 and over are eligible if they or their spouse have paid payroll taxes for 10 or more years. People under age 65 who are receiving disability benefits (SSI or SSDI) or who have end-stage renal disease or a diagnosis of ALS (Lou Gehrig's disease) are also eligible.

Medicare has four parts to its coverage:

- **Part A** – Hospital Insurance Program, which covers inpatient hospital services, skilled nursing facility, home health, and hospice care
- **Part B** – Supplementary Medical Insurance Program, which covers physician, outpatient, home health, and preventive services
- **Part C** – Medicare Advantage Program, which allows enrollment in private insurance plans
- **Part D** – Prescription drug benefit[24]

"Dual eligibles"—people over the age of 65 who are also low income—may qualify for both Medicare and Medicaid. In this case, Medicaid pays all of their Medicare premiums, deductibles, and co-pays and, importantly, pays for long-term care, such as nursing home care.

Children's Health Insurance Program

The Children's Health Insurance Program (CHIP), like Medicaid, is a health insurance program jointly funded by the federal government and the states. It provides coverage to uninsured children up to age 19 in families whose income is too high for them to qualify for Medicaid. States receive a federal match in funding based on the level at which they set eligibility for coverage. For example, if a state sets eligibility at 300% of the federal poverty level (FPL), its match will be higher than if it sets eligibility at 200% of the FPL. Generally, CHIP has been a popular program, garnering bipartisan support.[25] However, in 2017 Congress failed to fully renew funding for CHIP. As of the time of this writing, long-term funding for the program is uncertain.

Community Health Centers

Much of the discussion up to this point has been focused on how the government funds health insurance coverage for particular populations. But as you know, access to insurance does not always equal access to health care. As a result, the government also makes direct investments in health care delivery for low-income and medically needy individuals through community health centers (CHCs). CHCs provide primary health care to low-income and vulnerable patient populations across the U.S., regardless of ability to pay or insurance status. CHCs exist in all states and serve some 25 million people, or about 1 in 13 people in the U.S. One in six people on Medicaid and one in five uninsured people receive care at a CHC.[26]

Community health centers are organized as nonprofit clinics and are governed by four primary federal requirements. The health centers must: (1) be located in underserved areas and serve medically underserved populations; (2) provide comprehensive primary health care services; (3) operate on a sliding payment scale; and

(4) be governed by a community board from which the majority of members must be health center patients. Fifty-five percent of CHCs are located in rural areas and provide critical care to residents of underserved areas.[27] Because the Affordable Care Act increased direct funding to community health centers, they have been able to grow their services and the number of patients served, particularly in states that expanded their Medicaid programs. Medicaid payments make up 44% of revenue for CHCs.[28] Yet. funding for CHCs remains tenuous. As of late 2017, Congress has failed to reauthorize funding for CHCs and threats to federal Medicaid funding could significantly undermine the ability to deliver services.

Reproductive Health Care Services

The federal government provides funding for family planning and reproductive health care through Title X of the Public Health Service Act. Title X prioritizes funding for low-income and uninsured patients, with funding distributed to community-based hospitals, health centers, university health centers, and faith-based organizations. Services provided by Title X grantees include family planning, contraception, education and counseling, breast and pelvic cancer screening and exams, and screening and treatment of sexually transmitted diseases and HIV. Under the law, Title X funds may not be used for abortion services.

Planned Parenthood, a national family planning provider, receives approximately 25% of Title X funds. Because Planned Parenthood also offers abortion services (paid for by non–Title X funds), some policymakers have argued that Planned Parenthood should not receive any Title X funding. Cutting off Title X funding to clinics that also provide abortions could, however, have significant consequences for women's reproductive health care. A study by the Guttmacher Institute found that 15% of women in the U.S. receive their contraceptive prescriptions at Title X clinics, and 90% of those women also receive preventive gynecological care at the clinics. Fully 70% had incomes below the federal poverty level.[29]

In addition to the services provided by Title X, regulations passed by the U.S. Department of Health and Human Services (DHHS) under the Affordable Care Act include prescription contraception as part of a list of preventive services that must be covered—without any co-payments—by insurance policies. This contraceptive mandate has been controversial among religious conservatives who view the mandate as an attack on religious liberty. In response to concerns from religious organizations, the Obama Administration implemented an opt-out provision allowing insurance companies to provide contraceptive coverage without direct involvement from the religious organization. This compromise was rejected by some religious organizations, including the Conference of Catholic Bishops, which sued the federal government. In 2014, the Supreme Court ruled that the mandate violated closely held corporations' religious liberty rights under the federal Religious Freedom Restoration Act. (A closely held corporation is a company that has only a small number of shareholders, such as a family-owned company).[30] Additional challenges to the contraception mandate are still making their way through the courts. In October 2017, just before this book went into production, the Trump Administration issued two rules through DHHS, which offer an exemption to employers who claim religious or moral objection to covering contraception in their health insurance plans.[31]

▶ Food Assistance

As described in the chapter on social and structural barriers to health, food insecurity affects a significant segment of the U.S. population and has severe consequences for health, particularly for children. There are three main assistance programs designed to alleviate food insecurity and to support nutrition: the Supplemental Nutrition Assistance Program (SNAP), the Special Supplemental Nutrition Program for Women, Infants and Children (WIC), and the School Breakfast and School Lunch Programs.

Supplemental Nutrition Assistance Program

The Supplemental Nutrition Assistance Program (SNAP) (formerly called the Food Stamp Program) was originally created in 1939 as a way to promote the purchase of unmarketable farm surpluses by low-income populations. Over time, it has become the nation's most important antihunger program. SNAP is an entitlement program that provides monthly benefits through a set dollar amount for the purchase of qualifying foods. In 2016, SNAP accounted for 69% of all federal food and nutrition assistance spending, with an average of 44.2 million people participating in the program per month.[32] Nearly all low-income individuals are eligible for SNAP, though certain immigrants who are lawful permanent residents must undergo a waiting period before becoming eligible for benefits. Undocumented immigrants are not eligible. Childless unemployed adults are limited to receipt of the benefit for three months every three years. Under federal rules, states may waive the three-month limit during times of economic crisis. During the Great Recession many states suspended the time limit for single adults, but have since reinstated it as the economy has recovered.

The amount of the SNAP benefit depends on the size of a participating family and the family's income. Benefits are based on an assumption that families will spend 30% of their income on food. A family with no income would qualify for the maximum benefit, while a family with more income would receive the benefit calculated after their expected contribution. The average monthly benefit for a family of four in 2017 was $465.[33] While the federal government and states jointly fund the costs of administration of the SNAP program, the federal government is responsible for the full cost of SNAP benefits. At the federal level, SNAP is funded and administered through the U.S. Department of Agriculture (USDA)'s Food and Nutrition Service, which sets program guidelines and supports states in administering the program at the local level. States are responsible for conducting outreach and education, determining who is eligible, and distributing benefits. Hence, there is wide variance in uptake across states, with some states providing benefits to nearly all eligible individuals and families and other states reaching only a percentage of those eligible. Nationwide, it is estimated that about 16% of food-insecure households do not participate in the SNAP program.[34] Some of the gap in reaching eligible families may have to do with stigma associated with government assistance, but given that some states have much higher participation rates than others, outreach and education may also play a large role.

Because SNAP serves to reduce food insecurity and also acts as an income support, studies show that it significantly alleviates financial stress on families. Research by Shaefer and Gutierrez suggests that in addition to reducing food insecurity by 13%, SNAP also provides families with more resources for essential needs such as housing, utilities, and medical bills. They estimate that SNAP participation reduces the risk of falling behind on rent by 7%, while it reduces the risk of being unable to pay for utilities by 15%. SNAP appears to play a critical role in helping families to avoid the "heat or eat" dilemma described in the chapter on social and structural barriers to health. In addition, the researchers found that SNAP participation decreased the likelihood of forgoing medical care by 9%.[35]

The Special Supplemental Nutrition Program for Women, Infants and Children

The Special Supplemental Nutrition Program for Women, Infants and Children (WIC) is a federal program focused on protecting the nutritional health of pregnant or nursing women, infants, and children under age five. The eligibility requirements for participation in WIC are that the applicant must be:

- A resident in the state in which they are applying
- A pregnant or nursing woman, or a child under the age of five
- Low-income
- At risk for poor nutrition

While federal law sets the categorical eligibility requirements for the program (e.g., that the recipient be a qualifying woman, infant, or child), states have leeway in determining income thresholds for eligibility and nutritional requirements for determining if a recipient is "at risk for poor nutrition." Unlike SNAP, WIC does not have immigration status restrictions. Half of all American infants and a quarter of all children ages one to four are served by the WIC program. Mothers participating in WIC receive nutrition counseling, assistance with locating health care, and support with breastfeeding. Food packages are designed depending on the recipient (adult, infant, or child) and may include vouchers for cereal, milk, fresh produce, or formula.

A much smaller program than SNAP, WIC reaches roughly 7.7 million women and children and accounts for about $5.9 billion of the federal food assistance budget, while SNAP accounts for $70.8 billion.[36] Given the health consequences of poor nutrition for pregnant women and young children, WIC serves an important purpose in ensuring that nutritional needs are met during this critical period for mothers and young children. The evidence suggests that WIC improves health and well-being. One study assessing whether prenatal participation in WIC improved birth outcomes showed that it was associated with a significant reduction in the infant mortality rate among blacks.[37] Another study found that earlier and longer-term participation in WIC by mothers and children reduces food insecurity.[38]

The National School Lunch and Breakfast Programs

The National School Lunch Act was signed in 1946 by President Harry S. Truman to provide nutritious, low-cost or free meals to school-age children. The program now operates in more than 100,000 public schools, nonprofit private schools, and child care centers. Children in families with incomes below 130% of the federal poverty level are eligible for free lunch, while those from families with incomes between 130% and 185% of the poverty level are eligible for reduced-price lunch.

School meals must meet the nutrition standards set by the latest Dietary Guidelines for Americans. The Healthy Hunger-Free Kids Act of 2010 authorized funding and set policy for core child nutrition programs.[39] Under the Obama Administration, with leadership from First Lady Michelle Obama, federal standards were changed to increase fruits, vegetables, and whole grains in meals, to include calorie limits by age group, and to reduce sodium content. The stricter nutrition regulations met with significant criticism from school districts that complained that the guidelines were difficult to meet and that children were not eating and throwing away, the healthier meals. This criticism was echoed by Trump Administration Agriculture Secretary Sonny Perdue, who announced soon after taking office that the U.S. Department of Agriculture (USDA) would delay implementation of the sodium requirements and would allow waivers for the regulations regarding whole grains. Yet, evidence does not appear to support the claim that offering healthier meals to children is a waste. For example, a 2015 study published in *Childhood Obesity* found that students consumed more fruit and wasted less of their entrees and vegetables after revised nutritional standards went into effect.[40]

The School Breakfast Program (SBP) was established in 1966 to provide grants to schools to offer breakfast to "nutritionally needy" children. Initiated as a pilot program, schools located in poor areas or in areas where children had to travel a great distance to school were targeted for funding. In 1975, when the U.S. Congress made the program permanent, it continued to emphasize participation by schools with severe need. Similar to the School Lunch program, the program is governed by federal nutritional standards and eligibility requirements. Supporters of the SBP point to research documenting the relationship between hunger and poor academic achievement and the particular role that breakfast plays in improving cognition and attention in school.[41] In response to this argument, some school districts offer universal free breakfast, and some even provide it in the classroom rather than in the cafeteria to encourage all students to eat breakfast. A 2013 study by Mathematica Policy Research, a research foundation in Washington, DC, estimated the causal effects of universal free breakfast on academic achievement as measured by test scores. They posit that by reducing the stigma associated with only offering free breakfast to low-income children, students are more likely to participate. They found that improvements in test scores are "at least partly driven by year round benefits [of offering universal free breakfast] rather than only consumption at the time of testing."[42]

▶ Housing Assistance

Federal and state housing assistance programs for low-income individuals and families fall into two types of programs: public housing are units owned by housing authorities, usually administered at the state or local levels; the Section 8 voucher program allows eligible individuals and families to rent units in the private market using a subsidy provided by the housing authority. Both the public housing and Section 8 programs are overseen by the U.S. Department of Housing and Urban Development (HUD). Neither of these housing assistance programs are entitlements. Many states have lengthy waiting lists for eligible individuals and families, some as long as several years.[43] Due to limited funding, three out of four eligible families do not receive housing assistance and for "every assisted household in the United States, twice as many low-income households are homeless or pay more than half of their income for rent and do not receive any federal rental assistance."[44] Federal rules for eligibility are based on targeting the most needy: 75% of new households must be "extremely low income," meaning that its income cannot exceed 30% of the local median or the federal poverty level, whichever is higher. Generally, a family using a voucher must contribute either 30% of its income toward rent or a minimum rent of $50, depending on which is higher. Roughly a third of housing vouchers go to adults with children, about a quarter go to the elderly, and a fifth go to disabled adults.[45]

▶ The Justice System: Legal Protections That Address Social Determinants of Health

In addition to federal and state safety net programs intended to provide access to basic needs and promote health and well-being, the legal system provides certain protections for vulnerable populations that help to counter negative social and structural determinants of health. Below we summarize a selection of some key legal protections. It is not possible to fully outline legal protections related to all social and structural determinants of health here, but this discussion will provide you with an overview of some of the important ways that the law can support health and safety and strive to promote health justice. Like the many safety net programs that fall short in meeting the needs of eligible individuals and families, the legal system is often inadequate in enforcing the rights of low-income and disadvantaged people, rights that very often are important to protecting health and reducing disparities. As you read this section, ask yourself: how might the law be changed or how might existing laws be better enforced in order to foster health equity and justice?

The Justice Gap: Access to Legal Assistance for Low-Income People

Before highlighting legal rights associated with the health of vulnerable populations, it is first important to describe what is known as the "justice gap"—"the difference between the level of civil legal assistance available and the level that is necessary to meet the legal needs of low-income individuals and families."[46] Just as there is no right to health care in the U.S., there is no right to legal assistance in civil justice matters. Common civil legal problems affecting low-income individuals and families include wrongful denial of government benefits and entitlements, unlawful housing eviction, housing safety code violations, employment discrimination, and inadequate protection in cases of family violence. As we will discuss below, many of these problems strongly implicate individual and family health and well-being.

In 1974, Congress established the Legal Services Corporation, an independent nonprofit corporation that provides grants to state legal-aid organizations

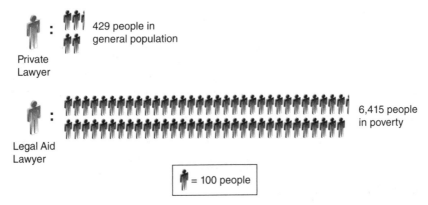

FIGURE 5.2 Comparison of private lawyers to general population and legal-aid lawyers to low-income population.

Legal Services Corporation. Documenting the justice gap in America: the current unmet civil legal needs of low-income Americans. September 2009.

to provide free legal assistance to qualifying low-income individuals, generally those whose incomes are below the federal poverty level. These include 133 non-profit legal-aid programs with 800 offices around the country. In addition to LSC-funded programs, there are legal-aid organizations that are funded through other means such as state and local governments, Interest on Lawyers' Trust Accounts (IOLTA), the private bar, and philanthropic foundations. As described in the chapter on health-harming legal doctrines, current funding for legal-aid programs is severely inadequate to meet the significant legal needs of low-income individuals and families. **FIGURE 5.2** shows how few legal-aid lawyers there are available to people living in poverty. Nearly a million individuals who seek out help with a civil legal problem are turned away due to lack of resources among legal-aid programs. A 2009 study by LSC found that 50% of those who sought legal assistance from an LSC-funded program were turned away. The lack of access to legal assistance has significant ramifications.[47] For example, a 2013 study in New York City found that 99% of tenants were unrepresented by legal counsel in housing eviction proceedings.[48]

Denial of Government Benefits and Entitlements

As described earlier, safety net programs provide crucial assistance to low-income people and help to reduce the number of people living in poverty. Because some safety net programs are legal entitlements—in other words, the government is obliged to provide the benefit to all who meet the eligibility requirements—eligible individuals who are wrongfully denied benefits or whose benefits are erroneously terminated may have legal recourse. An eligible individual may be denied a benefit for a number of reasons: administrative error, communication problems between a government agency and the recipient, or confusion about changing eligibility standards. Often it is difficult for individuals, especially those living in poverty, to have the time, resources, and knowledge to challenge a government bureaucracy's decision on his or her own. As noted earlier, for some government benefits, such as disability income (SSI), initial denials and delays are common.

Denial of income supports, health insurance, or food assistance can have devastating effects on individuals and families who are living below or close to the poverty line. Lawyers who know the rules and eligibility requirements for these programs can challenge erroneous denials and help to restore benefits before individuals and families are seriously harmed. But because of the scarcity of free legal assistance available to low-income people, many go without legal help in these matters.

Laws Protecting Housing Stability and Safety
Eviction

As described in the chapter on social and structural barriers to health, eviction from housing is extremely common for low-income individuals and families and has important health consequences, particularly for low-income mothers and children. Because many low-income tenants do not have written tenancy agreements or leases, they have few protections from eviction. In most states, tenants must be provided with adequate notice before they may be lawfully evicted. This time period usually conforms to how the tenant pays his or her rent. For example, if tenant pays rent on a monthly basis, he or she must be given 30-days' notice before he or she may be evicted without cause. However, if the tenant violates the state's tenancy laws by, for example, failing to pay his or her rent on time, he or she may be evicted lawfully through a court process set by law.

Because many low-income tenants are evicted for nonpayment of rent, they often have no legal recourse. In this case, if the landlord follows the appropriate process for evicting the tenant, he or she has the right to do so. However, sometimes a tenant may have a defense or counterclaim in an eviction proceeding. For example, if a landlord fails to meet his or her responsibilities under housing health and safety laws, a tenant may use this as a defense to eviction and make a counterclaim against the landlord for failing to meet his or her duty. Unfortunately, many low-income tenants are unaware of their legal rights or are unable to obtain legal assistance. As noted above, a study in New York found that 99% of tenants are unrepresented in eviction proceedings.[49] Because of the lack of access to legal assistance, most low-income tenants are at a severe disadvantage in protecting their legal rights.

Housing Maintenance and Safety Codes

Tenants also have the legal right to live in a property that does not endanger their health or safety. States and municipalities have housing maintenance and safety laws, usually referred to as the "housing code," that spell out housing conditions that endanger health and safety and that, therefore, violate the code. Most states and localities have agencies that inspect properties for housing health and safety violations. If a tenant believes that a property is in violation of the housing code, he or she may contact this agency and request an inspection. If the inspection determines that a property is in violation of the code, a landlord is sent a notice of violation and given a specified period of time to correct the violation(s). If he or she fails to do so, he or she may be fined.

Low-income tenants face a number of problems enforcing their legal right to safe housing. First, many low-income tenants are unaware of their rights or, if they are, they may not know how to exercise those rights. In most jurisdictions the burden is on a tenant to complain to the appropriate housing code enforcement agency and seek an inspection of the property. For vulnerable tenants who have poor bargaining power and few affordable housing options, the risk of antagonizing a landlord, who may resort to eviction in retaliation for alerting authorities, is often not in their best interest. While many states have laws protecting tenants from retaliatory eviction, these laws frequently go unenforced. Second, because many housing code agencies are underresourced and/or poorly administered, the responses to tenant complaints are often discretionary and inadequate. Legal assistance can help vulnerable tenants enforce their rights. Another option is for cities to implement proactive enforcement in which cities target particular areas for routine inspections based on the likelihood of housing code violations. This approach removes the burden of enforcing their own rights from vulnerable tenants, and creates a more systematic way for cities to ensure that housing remains safe.[50]

Employment Protections

While it is beyond the scope of this chapter to outline all of the legal protections available to workers, we focus on three that specifically implicate health and safety.

Workers' Compensation

A state-mandated insurance program, Workers' Compensation provides compensation to workers for job-related illnesses and injuries. Workers' Compensation is a no-fault program, meaning that workers are eligible for compensation, regardless of who is at fault for the injury. Workers compensated under the program relinquish their right to sue the employer for damages based on their injuries. Unfortunately, the Workers' Compensation system appears to be failing most low-wage workers. A 2009 study of violations of labor laws in American cities found that of the workers surveyed who had been seriously injured in their jobs, only 8% had filed a Workers' Compensation claim, and of all the injured workers in the sample, only 6% ultimately had claims paid through Workers' Compensation. Fifty percent of individuals who told their employer of their injury experienced an illegal response from their employer—"including firing the worker, calling immigration authorities, or instructing the worker not to file for Workers' Compensation."[51]

The Americans with Disabilities Act

The Americans with Disabilities Act (ADA) prohibits discrimination on the basis of disability in employment (among other things). The ADA defines a disabled person as someone who has:

- A physical or mental impairment that substantially limits a major life activity
- A history of such a disability (such as cancer in remission)
- Is regarded as having a disability (even if he or she doesn't)

Notwithstanding the ADA, disabled employees must still be able to perform the essential functions of their job with or without reasonable accommodations, and they must be able to satisfy the employer's requirements for the job—e.g., education level, skills, and past experience. The ADA permits qualifying disabled employees to seek a reasonable accommodation that will allow them to perform their jobs, though the request may not entail a fundamental alteration of the job or workplace and the accommodation may not cause "undue hardship" to the employer. A reasonable accommodation includes any change to a job, work environment, or the way a job is typically done to allow a person with a disability to apply for the job, perform the job duties, and have equal access to benefits available to other employees.[52]

The goal of the ADA is to ensure that people with disabilities do not face discrimination in the workplace and are not excluded from employment. An employee may have a legal claim under the ADA if his or her employer discriminates against him or her based on disability or if it refuses to provide a reasonable accommodation as permitted by the law. Given the importance of employment to health, the ADA plays an important role in protecting the jobs and well-being of disabled employees.

The Family and Medical Leave Act

The Family and Medical Leave Act (FMLA) provides up to 12 weeks of unpaid, job-protected leave to qualifying employees for specified circumstances. These include:

- The birth or adoption of a child
- To care for a seriously ill family member (spouse, child, or parent)
- To care for an injured service member in the family or in some cases for circumstances arising out a family member's deployment
- To recover from the employee's own illness

The law covers government employers, schools, and private sector employers who employee 50 or more workers. To qualify, an employee must have been employed for at least 12 months and have worked at least 1,250 hours during the previous year. Employees do not have to take all 12 weeks of leave at once; it may be used on an intermittent basis as long as it meets the requirements of the law.[53]

The law applies to only about one in six worksites in the U.S. because smaller employers are exempted and it excludes roughly half of employees based on its hourly requirements.[54] Furthermore, while the law protects employees from losing their jobs because of the need to take time off for illness or to care for a family member, it does not require that the employer pay the employee during his or her absence. For low-income workers who are not in a position to take unpaid leave, the law may have little value. Most low-income mothers do not get paid when they need to care for a sick child. This includes two-thirds of women with income below 200% of the federal poverty level and three-quarters of women living below poverty.[55] While 10% of workers earning more than $65,000 per year lack access to paid sick leave, nearly 80% of workers earning less than $15,000 per year do; low-wage workers are also less likely to have access to paid family leave.[56]

Lack of access to paid sick and family leave has important implications for health. It puts low-income families in an untenable position of choosing between foregoing income for basic needs, potentially losing employment altogether, or taking needed time during illness or to care for a sick family member. Increasingly, states and some counties and cities are passing paid sick and family leave laws. In the three states that currently have paid family leave laws (California, Rhode Island, and

New Jersey), the programs are funded through employee-paid payroll taxes and are administered through the state's disability insurance program.[57]

Protections for Victims of Intimate Partner Violence and Child Maltreatment

As described in the chapter on social and structural barriers to health, family violence can take a large toll on the physical and mental health of adult and child victims. The legal system's primary tool for protecting victims from future abuse is the civil protection order (often referred to as a restraining order or no-contact order), which legally bars the perpetrator from contacting or coming within a designated distance from the victim. These orders may also include that the perpetrator stay away from the victim's children. The Violence Against Women Act of 2000, a federal law, provides grants to support legal assistance to victims in obtaining these orders.

Civil protection orders are intended to prevent any future abuse and harassment by the perpetrator. While they are an important tool in providing safety for victims and their children, studies suggest that nearly 50% of civil protection orders are violated at least once.[58] It is important to acknowledge that protective orders and the legal system are only part of providing safety from intimate partner violence (IPV). Because perpetrators of IPV seek power and control over the victim, his or her use of the legal system to regain control may actually incite more violence and danger. Careful safety planning should include ensuring that the victim and his or her children have a safe location to which to relocate, if necessary. Because low-income victims are less likely to have the financial means to relocate, they may require comprehensive supports, such as housing assistance and income supports to be able to fully separate from an abuser.

It is also important to note that when the victim of IPV has children with the abuser, permanent separation is even more difficult. Courts are loath to completely terminate a parent's right to contact with his or her children, particularly if the parent has not directly abused the child. It is common for a perpetrator of IPV to use the legal process as an opportunity to continue to harass, threaten, and abuse the victim parent. As research continues to demonstrate the detrimental effects on children of exposure to violence in the home, courts have increasingly taken into account a history of IPV in custody decisions and visitation arrangements. However, it is rare for a parent who has engaged in IPV to have visitation terminated altogether. In making custody and visitation decisions, courts generally apply the "best interests of the child" standard, weighing a list of factors to determine the frequency of contact between each parent and the child. Legal advocates and health care providers play a key role in informing the court about the effects of past violence on children, as well as the risk of future exposure after divorce or separation.

When a child has been maltreated by a parent, an entirely different legal process is used. Each state has its own laws that define abuse and neglect and determine who is obligated to report child abuse and neglect, as well as the designated agency that will receive reports and investigate them. Most state laws require certain professionals to report suspected abuse or neglect when acting in their professional capacity. These generally include physicians, nurses, social workers, teachers, and child care providers. Some states require that any person who suspects child abuse or neglect to report it.

The government agency responsible for investigating child abuse, usually referred to as "Child Protective Services" (CPS), has the authority to determine if there is credible evidence supporting the allegation of abuse and what further action will be taken. Typically, once a report is made to the agency, it investigates to determine if a case should be opened or if the report does not warrant further action. Once a case is opened, the agency may petition the court to have the child temporarily removed from the home and placed in foster care or if it determines that the child is not in immediate danger, it may allow the child to remain in the home with agency oversight and services to the family. State laws and policies set timelines for each stage of the process. Concerned that too many children were lingering for long periods of time in foster care, Congress passed the Adoption and Safe Families Act of 1997 to specify that CPS agencies must make reasonable efforts to keep the child in the home safely. If the child is removed from the home, the agency must create a permanency plan and a review hearing must be held within 12 months of the child being removed from the home, at which time the child may be reunified with his or her family or the agency will file for a termination of parental rights in order to place the child in an adoptive home.[59]

Despite efforts to improve the child welfare system by putting pressure on CPS agencies to move children out of the system more quickly, significant problems remain. Lawyers working on child welfare cases cite a laundry list of problems: lack of basic services for vulnerable families, inadequacy of mental health services for children and parents, lack of preventive services to reduce involvement with the system in the first place, and issues with the CPS workforce including lack of training, high caseloads and turnover, and difficulty recruiting foster parents.[60]

▶ Conclusion

The story of America's safety net and legal protections for vulnerable populations is a mixed one. On the one hand, safety net programs are critically important in helping vulnerable individuals and families live above the federal poverty level and to have access to health care, nutritious food, and housing. On the other hand, many safety net programs reach only a portion of the people who need them and are not always sufficient to truly protect health and well-being. Some eligible individuals and families are wrongfully denied services or benefits and have little legal recourse. Recall, as was discussed earlier, the U.S. invests substantially less than other comparable countries in social supports and has worse health outcomes. In fact, one study predicted that life expectancy in the U.S. would increase by 3.77 years "if it had just the average social policy generosity of the other 17 [Organisation for Economic Co-operation and Development (OECD)] nations."[61]

Similarly, legal protections intended to protect people from homelessness, unsafe housing, employment discrimination and job loss, and family violence often go unenforced, particularly for low-income people. The justice gap places an enormous burden on low-income individuals to know about and attempt to enforce their legal rights on their own, without the assistance of lawyers. Because employment and income, and access to nutritious food, safe and affordable housing, and freedom from exposure to violence are all critical to health, ensuring that individuals and families have the social supports and the ability to exercise their legal rights plays a major role in health justice. Yet, the debate about who is deserving of government assistance, how much support should be afforded, and the role of the federal government in funding safety net and legal assistance programs continues to rage on.

References

1. Ryan AM, Dacchille C, Wolf DF, Lawton E. Income and health: dynamics of employment and the safety net. In: Tobin Tyler E, Lawton E, Conroy C, Sandel M, et al., eds. *Poverty, Health and Law: Readings and Cases for Medical-Legal Partnership*. Durham, NC: Carolina Academic Press; 2012: 192–193.
2. Irving SK, Loveless TA. Dynamics of economic well-being: participation in government programs, 2009–2012: who gets assistance? United States Census Bureau; May 2015. Available at: https://www.census.gov/content/dam/Census/library/publications/2015/demo/p70-141.pdf. Accessed October 10, 2017.
3. Irving SK, Loveless TA. Dynamics of economic well-being: participation in government programs, 2009–2012: who gets assistance? United States Census Bureau; May 2015. Available at: https://www.census.gov/content/dam/Census/library/publications/2015/demo/p70-141.pdf. Accessed October 10, 2017.
4. The Personal Responsibility and Work Opportunity Reconciliation Act, Pub. L. 104–193; Center for Budget and Policy Priorities. An introduction to TANF; June 15, 2015. Available at: https://www.cbpp.org/research/policy-basics-an-introduction-to-tanf. Accessed October 10, 2017.
5. Stanley M, Floyd I. TANF cash benefits have fallen by more than 20 percent in most states and continue to erode. Center for Budget and Policy Priorities; October 17, 2016. Available at: https://www.cbpp.org/research/family-income-support/tanf-cash-benefits-have-fallen-by-more-than-20-percent-in-most-states. Accessed October 10, 2017.
6. The World Bank. Poverty. Available at: www.worldbank.org/en/topic/poverty/overview. Accessed January 10, 2018.
7. Floyd I, Pavetti L, Schott, L. TANF reaching few poor families. Center for Budget and Policy Priorities; March 20, 2017. Available at: https://www.cbpp.org/research/family-income-support/tanf-reaching-few-poor-families. Accessed October 10, 2017.
8. Renzulli, KA. This is how much the average American spends on child care. *Time*. August 9, 2016. Available at: http://time.com/money/4444034/average-cost-child-care/. Accessed October 10, 2017.
9. Minton S, Durham C. Low-income families and the cost of child care: state child care subsidies, out-of-pocket expenses, and the cliff effect. Urban Institute; December 2013:1. Availave at https://www.urban.org/research/publication/low-income-families-and-cost-child-care. Accessed February 22, 2018.
10. National Women's Law Center (NWLC). Temporary assistance for needy families and child care assistance: a weakened safety net for families; November 2016. Available at: https://nwlc.org/wp-content/uploads/2016/11/TANF-Child-Care-Fact-Sheet-11.4.16.pdf. Accessed October 10, 2017.
11. National Women's Law Center (NWLC). Temporary assistance for needy families and child care assistance: a weakened safety net for families; November 2016. Available at: https://nwlc.org/wp-content/uploads/2016/11/TANF-Child-Care-Fact-Sheet-11.4.16.pdf. Accessed October 10, 2017.
12. Mather A. Childcare costs: yet another way we're failing the poor. *Forbes*. February 1, 2016. Available at: https://www.forbes.com/sites/aparnamathur/2016/02/01/childcare-costs-yet-another-way-were-failing-the-poor/2/#21c93a9427bd. Accessed January 11, 2018.
13. Duncan GJ, Magnuson K. Investing in preschool programs. *The Journal of Economic Perspectives: A Journal of the American Economic Association*. Spring 2013;27(2):109–132.
14. Votruba-Drzal E, Coley RL, Maldonado-Carreño C, et al. Child care and the development of behavior problems among economically disadvantaged children in middle childhood. *Child Development*. 2010;81(5):1460–1474.
15. Centers for Disease Control and Prevention. Disability impacts all of us. Available at: https://www.cdc.gov/ncbddd/disabilityandhealth/infographic-disability-impacts-all.html. Accessed October 10, 2017.

16. Social Security Administration. Code of Federal Regulations. §416.926a. Functional equivalence for children.

17. Autor DH. The unsustainable rise of the disability rolls in the United States: causes, consequences, and policy options. MIT and National Bureau of Economic Research; November 23, 2011. Available at: https://economics.mit.edu/files/11610.

18. Ryan AM, Dacchille C, Wolf DF, Lawton E. Income and health: dynamics of employment and the safety net. In: Tobin Tyler E, Lawton E, Conroy C, Sandel M, et al., eds. *Poverty, Health and Law: Readings and Cases for Medical-Legal Partnership*. Durham, NC: Carolina Academic Press; 2012: 192–193.

19. Boone C, Dube A, Goodman L, Kaplan E. Unemployment insurance extension during great recession did not destroy jobs. Institute for New Economic Thinking; October 13, 2016. Available at: https://www.ineteconomics.org/perspectives/blog/unemployment-insurance -extension-during-great-recession-did-not-destroy-jobs. Accessed January 11, 2018.

20. Center for Budget and Policy Priorities. Policy basics: the earned income tax credit; October 21, 2016. Available at: https://www.cbpp.org/research/federal-tax/policy-basics-the-earned -income-tax-credit. Accessed January 11, 2018.

21. National Federation of Independent Business v. Sebelius, 567 U.S. 519 (2012).

22. The Henry J. Kaiser Family Foundation. Status of state action on the Medicaid expansion decision; January 1, 2017. Available at: https://www.kff.org/health-reform/state-indicator /state-activity-around-expanding-medicaid-under-the-affordable-care-act/?currentTime frame=0&sortModel=%7B%22colId%22:%22Location%22,%22sort%22:%22asc%22%7D. Accessed January 11, 2018.

23. The Henry J. Kaiser Family Foundation. Medicaid Pocket Primer; June 9, 2017. Available at: https://www.kff.org/medicaid/fact-sheet/medicaid-pocket-primer/. Accessed January11, 2018.

24. The Henry J. Kaiser Family Foundation. An overview of Medicare; April 1, 2016. Available at: https://www.kff.org/medicare/issue-brief/an-overview-of-medicare/. Accessed January11, 2018.

25. Children's Health Insurance Program. Medicaid.gov. Available at: https://www.medicaid.gov /chip/index.html https://www.medicaid.gov/chip/index.html. Accessed January11, 2018.

26. National Association of Community Health Centers. Strengthening the safety net: community health centers on the front lines of American health care; March 2017. Available at: http://www .nachc.org/wp-content/uploads/2017/03/Strengthening-the-Safety-Net_NACHC_2017.pdf.

27. National Association of Community Health Centers. Strengthening the safety net: community health centers on the front lines of American health care; March 2017. Available at: http://www .nachc.org/wp-content/uploads/2017/03/Strengthening-the-Safety-Net_NACHC_2017.pdf.

28. National Association of Community Health Centers. Strengthening the safety net: community health centers on the front lines of American health care; March 2017. Available at: http://www .nachc.org/wp-content/uploads/2017/03/Strengthening-the-Safety-Net_NACHC_2017.pdf.

29. National Public Radio. At-risk federal funds cover far more than the pill; April 1, 2011. Available at: http://www.npr.org/2011/04/01/135018313/at-risk-federal-funds-cover-far-more-than-the -pill. Accessed January11, 2018.

30. Burwell v. Hobby Lobby Stores, 573 US ___ (2014).

31. Pear R, Ruiz RR, Goodstein L. Trump administration rolls back birth control mandate. *The New York Times*. October 6, 2017. Available at: https://www.nytimes.com/2017/10/06/us /politics/trump-contraception-birth-control.html. Accessed January 11, 2018.

32. Oliveira V. The food assistance landscape: FY 2016 Annual Report. U.S. Department of Agriculture; March 2017. Available at: https://www.ers.usda.gov/webdocs/publications/82994 /eib169_summary.pdf?v=42823.

33. Center for Budget and Policy Priorities. A quick guide to SNAP eligibility and benefits; September 14, 2017. Available at: https://www.cbpp.org/research/a-quick-guide-to-snap -eligibility-and-benefits. Accessed January 11, 2018.

34. Whitmore DS, Bauer L, Nantz G. Twelve facts about food insecurity and SNAP. Brookings Institution; April 21, 2016. Available at: https://www.brookings.edu/research /twelve-facts-about-food-insecurity-and-snap/.

35. Shaefer HL, Gutierrez IA. The Supplemental Nutrition Assistance Program and material hardships among low-income households with children. *Social Service Review.* December 2013;87(4):753–779.

36. Carlson S, Neuberger Z, Rosenbaum D. WIC participation and costs are unstable. Center for Budget and Policy Priorities; July 19, 2017. Available at: https://www.cbpp.org/research/food -assistance/wic-participation-and-costs-are-stable. Accessed January 11, 2018.

37. Khanani I, Elam J, Hearn R, et al. The impact of prenatal WIC participation on infant mortality and racial disparities. *American Journal of Public Health.* April 2010;100(Suppl 1):S204–S209.

38. Metallinos-Katsaras E, Gorman KS, Wilde P, Kallio J. A longitudinal study of WIC participation on household food insecurity. *Maternal and Child Health Journal.* July 2011;15(5):627–633.

39. U.S. Department of Agriculture. School meals: Healthy Hunger-Free Kids Act. Available at: https:// www.fns.usda.gov/school-meals/healthy-hunger-free-kids-act. Accessed January 11, 2018.

40. Marlene B. Schwartz MB, Henderson KE, et al. New school meal regulations increase fruit consumption and do not increase total plate waste. *Childhood Obesity.* June 2015;11(3):242–247.

41. Food Action and Research Center. Research brief: breakfast for learning; October 2016. Available at: http://frac.org/wp-content/uploads/breakfastforlearning-1.pdf.

42. Dotter DD. Breakfast at the desk: the impact of universal breakfast programs on academic performance. Mathematica Policy Research; October 2013. Available at: http://www.appam .org/assets/1/7/Breakfast_at_the_Desk_The_Impact_of_Universal_Breakfast_Programs_on _Academic_Performance.pdf.

43. Center for Budget and Policy Priorities. Policy basics: federal rental assistance; May 3, 2017. Available at: https://www.cbpp.org/research/housing/policy-basics-federal-rental-assistance. Accessed January 11, 2018.

44. Center for Budget and Policy Priorities. United States: Fact sheet: federal rental assistance; March 30, 2017. Available at: https://www.cbpp.org/sites/default/files/atoms/files/4-13 -11hous-US.pdf.

45. Center for Budget and Policy Priorities. Who is helped by housing choice vouchers? Available at: www.cbpp.org/who-is-helped-by-housing-choice-vouchers-0. Accessed on January 11, 2018.

46. Legal Services Corporation. The unmet need for legal aid. Available at: http://www.lsc.gov /what-legal-aid/unmet-need-legal-aid. Accessed January 11, 2018.

47. Legal Services Corporation. Documenting the justice gap in America: the current unmet civil legal needs of low-income Americans; September 2009. Available at: https://www.americanbar .org/content/dam/aba/migrated/marketresearch/PublicDocuments/JusticeGaInAmerica2009. authcheckdam.pdf.

48. Legal Services Corporation. The unmet need for legal aid. Available at: http://www.lsc.gov /what-legal-aid/unmet-need-legal-aid. Accessed January 11, 2018.

49. Legal Services Corporation. The unmet need for legal aid. Available at: http://www.lsc.gov /what-legal-aid/unmet-need-legal-aid. Accessed January 11, 2018.

50. Change Lab Solutions. Healthy housing through proactive rental inspection; 2014. Available at: http://www.changelabsolutions.org/sites/default/files/Healthy_Housing_Proactive_Rental _Inspection_FINAL_20140421.pdf.

51. Bernhardt A, Milkman R, Theodore N, et al. Broken laws, unprotected workers: violation of employment and labor laws in America's cities; 2009. Available at: http://www.nelp.org /content/uploads/2015/03/BrokenLawsReport2009.pdf?nocdn=1.

52. U.S. Department of Labor. The Americans with Disabilities Act. Available at: https://www.dol .gov/odep/topics/ADA.htm. Accessed January 11, 2018.

53. U.S. Department of Labor. Family and Medical Leave Act (FMLA). Available at: https://www .dol.gov/general/topic/benefits-leave/fmla. Accessed January 11, 2018.

54. Abt Associates. Family and medical leave in 2012. Report for the U.S. Department of Labor; September 13, 2013. Available at: https://www.dol.gov/asp/evaluation/fmla/FMLA-2012 -Executive-Summary.pdf.

55. Ben-Ishai L. Wages lost, jobs at risk: the serious consequences of lack of paid leave. Center for Law and Social Policy; February 5, 2015. Available at: http://www.clasp.org/resources-and -publications/publication-1/2015-02-03-FMLA-Anniversary-Brief.pdf.

56. National Partnership for Women and Families. Paid sick days – state, district and county statutes; updated November 2016. Available at: http://www.nationalpartnership.org/research -library/work-family/psd/paid-sick-days-statutes.pdf.

57. National Partnership for Women and Families. Paid sick days – state, district and county statutes; updated November 2016. Available at: http://www.nationalpartnership.org /research-library/work-family/psd/paid-sick-days-statutes.pdf; National Conference of State Legislatures. State family and medical leave laws; July 19, 2016. Available at: http://www.ncsl .org/research/labor-and-employment/state-family-and-medical-leave-laws.aspx.

58. McAlister Groves B, Pilnik L, Tobin Tyler E, et al. Personal safety: addressing interpersonal and family violence in the health and legal systems. In: Tobin Tyler E, Lawton E, Conroy C, Sandel M, et al., eds. *Poverty, Health and Law: Readings and Cases for Medical-Legal Partnership.* Durham, NC: Carolina Academic Press; 2012: 359.

59. The Adoption and Safe Families Act of 1997. PL 105-89. Available at: https://www.gpo.gov /fdsys/pkg/PLAW-105publ89/pdf/PLAW-105publ89.pdf.

60. National Association of Counsel for Children. Asking the experts: what are the three most critical issues facing child welfare today? Available at: https://www.naccchildlawblog.org /child-welfare-law/asking-the-experts-what-are-the-three-most-critical-issues-facing-child -welfare-today/. Accessed January 11, 2018.

61. Beckfield J, Bambra C. Shorter lives in stingier states: social policy shortcomings help explain the US mortality disadvantage. *Social Science & Medicine.* 2016;171:30–38.

CHAPTER 6

Systems Change to Promote Health Equity

LEARNING OBJECTIVES

By the end of this chapter you will be able to:

- Explain how some recent health care system reforms may support health justice.
- Describe initiatives focused on aligning health care, public health, social and legal services.
- Discuss federal, state, and local cross-sector policy efforts designed to address the social determinants of health.
- Assess educational reforms intended to improve interprofessional education about health justice.

▶ Introduction

The growing attention to social determinants of health (SDOH) and to the disconnect between the health care system and community-based resources is leading to new health care delivery system reforms, public health interventions, and intersectoral partnerships focused on improving population health. Many of these efforts have been guided and supported by the Affordable Care Act (ACA), which, in addition to expanding access to health care to individuals who historically were viewed as "uninsurable," promotes payment reforms and population health-focused initiatives that encourage a more holistic approach to health. In this chapter, we explore some of these reforms and initiatives with an eye toward how effectively they address SDOH and move the country further along the path to health justice. One lesson that has already been learned is that the health care and public health systems cannot do this on their own. Because health care makes up a relatively small percentage of a person's ability to get and stay healthy, the communities and systems with which people interact must also support health. And, for communities and systems to foster health, local, state, and federal policies and funding priorities must explicitly pay attention to population health. We have divided this chapter into five main parts to explore different approaches to improving population health and promoting health justice: (1) health care system reforms; (2) aligning health care, public health, and social services; (3) moving upstream: federal, state, and local initiatives; (4) linking health, law, and justice; and (5) the next generation: education for change. As you read this chapter, consider how laws and policies shape the ways in which health care is delivered to vulnerable populations, as well as how they support or undermine health equity and justice. Additionally, think about upstream and downstream approaches to health equity: what policy and systems changes are most likely to have the greatest impact on population health?

▶ Health Care System Reforms That Support Vulnerable Patients and Populations

In 2008, Donald M. Berwick, Thomas W. Nolan, and John Whittington published an article in *Health Affairs* in which they coined the term "the triple aim" of health care reform. In the article, they set out three simultaneous goals for health care reform: "improving the experience of care, improving the health of populations, and reducing per capita costs of health care."[1] To be successful, they argued, a health care organization must accept responsibility for all three goals for the population that it serves. Since 2008, the idea that health care organizations and providers are responsible not just for individual patients, but for population health outcomes, has become widely accepted, particularly in the delivery of primary care. The integration of a population health focus into health care has led to a whole host of reforms to health care delivery. These include: a push toward understanding the root causes of illness; preventing illness and promoting wellness, rather than focusing on care once people get sick; attempts to coordinate care across a siloed and fragmented health care system to not only improve the experience of care, but also to reduce unnecessary health care costs; use of data to track patient and population health outcomes; restructuring payment for health care services away from fee-for-service (i.e., paying by the visit or procedure) toward value-based payment (centered on effective management of a population of patients); and efforts to identify and address SDOH that drive poor health outcomes, health disparities, and higher health care costs.[2]

One of the driving forces that initially led stakeholders to focus on SDOH as a part of health care is data from the last two decades demonstrating escalating costs associated with chronic disease management. As alluded to in this text's Introduction, the United States has a higher burden of chronic disease than 16 peer nations for conditions including diabetes, obesity, chronic lung disease, heart disease, and disability.[3] Indeed, total spending in the Medicare program in 2010 was $300 billion, nearly all of which supported people with two or more chronic diseases.[4] Chronic disease is not disbursed equally among the population. As we have highlighted in other chapters, people with lower socioeconomic status, racial and ethnic minorities, and people in disadvantaged communities have a higher burden of chronic disease. Therefore, the cost of chronic disease management and the disparities associated with it have helped to fuel innovations in the health care system aimed at improving the health (and reducing the cost of care) for vulnerable populations.

Payment Reforms and Integrated Care Models: Opportunities to Foster Health Equity

The paradox in the U.S.—that it spends enormously on health care while having comparatively poor population health outcomes—has shined a light on how the nation pays for health care services, as well as how costs are distributed across patient populations. The U.S. approach to health care spending has largely been driven by a "fee-for-service" model: health care providers are either paid directly by patients at the time of treatment or reimbursed by a patient's health insurance company for each individual service rendered. Imagine a hospital bill for a patient who has just received a hip replacement, for example. Under a fee-for-service model, each inter-action with a health care provider (e.g., the surgeon, anesthesiologist, nurse), each medication, each bandage used for the dressing would be itemized separately on the bill, often at significant administrative cost. While a patient may not be responsible for these costs because he or she has insurance, they are costs to the system, nonetheless. Health care reformers have pointed out that fee for service payment incentivizes providers and hospitals to provide as many services as possible, rather than focus on the necessity and effectiveness of the procedure in making the patient healthier.

Following the triple aim goals of improving care, lowering costs, and promoting better population health outcomes, reformers have supported shifting to a value-based payment model. Value is essentially defined as "the quality of care (the sum of outcomes, safety, and service) divided by the cost of care over time."[5] Value-based payment is generally achieved through some sort of "bundled" or "global" payment mechanism, rather than through the traditional fee-for-service model. A bundled payment is episode based. For example, a provider is paid a lump sum (bundled payment) to cover the costs of a patient's hip replacement surgery. A global payment is made to a provider or group of providers to cover all of the costs of caring for a particular patient. The idea is to incentivize providers to use health care resources wisely and efficiently. The "value" in value-based payment models is measured by patient outcomes data, patient experience and quality metrics, and demonstration of reduced costs for caring for the population of patients over time. In return, the providers can expect that the payer (most often, thus far, the government through Medicare or Medicaid, or perhaps a private insurance company that has adopted value-based purchasing) will share with them the savings created by a more efficient and high-quality delivery of care.

The primary organizational model for value-based payment is the account-able care organization (ACO). ACOs are organizations that coordinate care among a group of health care providers (e.g., primary care practices, hospitals), which together manage the care for a defined population of patients and are held accountable for the quality of care, costs, and outcomes of that population. ACOs utilize a value-based purchasing model, most often a "capitated" model in which the ACO receives a per-patient, per-month payment to care for its designated population. Generally, ACOs share the financial risk of providing care with the government (Medicare and Medicaid) or an insurance company by contracting upfront to meet specific quality measures and cost targets. If those targets are met, the ACO providers are rewarded with a bonus payment; if not, they may be financially penalized.

You may be wondering at this point: how do these payment reforms and ACOs relate to health equity and justice? While not explicitly focused on health equity, the ACO model has forced health care organizations and insurance providers to pay attention to health disparities in a number of ways. First, while capitated payment models, such as the per-patient, per-month model, may suggest that all patients are roughly equal in health care needs and costs, clearly they are not. Healthier patients require less care, while sicker patients—particularly those with chronic disease(s)—may require a far more significant amount of care. Consider this:

> Roughly one half of patients in a primary care population are healthy (bottom of the pyramid) and constitute 10 percent to 20 percent of the total health care dollars spent. Thirty to 45 percent of the population has limited and/or stable chronic disease; the cost of caring for this group is roughly 30 percent to 40 percent of total costs. The sickest patients are in the smallest percentage (5 percent) of the population and are often described as [high-need, high-cost patients]. They often are elderly, frail, disadvantaged socioeconomically, have psychosocial barriers to care, and have multiple health issues and/or many emergency department visits and hospitalizations. They account for 45 to 50 percent of the health care costs in a population.[6]

To be effective in meeting quality, cost, and outcome measures, an ACO must pay close attention not only to the health care needs of their population, but also to how it can better coordinate care across systems and address nonmedical and social needs that may be leading to health care overutilization. It also must show better outcomes for its entire patient population, something that was not measured under the old fee-for-service payment model.

Second, payment reforms have helped to initiate discussion about "risk stratification." Risk stratification is a method of identifying patients who may require more care based on a particular characteristic. For example, a patient with poorly managed diabetes is at higher risk for complications (and potential visits to the emergency room or hospital) than a patient with well-managed diabetes. When health care providers are engaged in risk management through a value-based payment model, they are incentivized to track their patients in order to most effectively manage their care and reduce unnecessary spending. Since the burden of chronic disease is not equal among different groups, risk stratification can help lead to best practices for caring for vulnerable patient populations. In addition, given that SDOH can drive poor health outcomes and higher health care costs, reformers are promoting the incorporation of social determinants into risk stratification algorithms, allowing for increased reimbursement for care of particularly vulnerable patient populations.[7] Later in this chapter, we will describe some of the ways that risk stratification is being used to design interventions that address the social needs of complex patients.

Finally, value-based payment models have supported a shift in focus from the individual patient in the exam room to the needs of the population living in the community. Rather than focus solely on the personal attributes of an individual patient, health care providers are being asked to think about all of the upstream factors that influence their patients' health; this inevitably leads them to a better understanding of SDOH. It also requires them to think differently about what a patient may need to improve his or her health, well beyond biomedical remedies. Perhaps most importantly, it has provoked health care system redesign, disrupting the one patient–one doctor arrangements of the past to make way for a team approach to health care.

Integrated and Team-Based Care Models

To address the enormous problem of fragmentation in the health care system—in other words, the problem of focusing on various parts of an individual in search of a "cure" or remedy without adequately appreciating the totality of the person and the person's life circumstances—several models of care integration have taken shape in the past two decades. Here we will focus on models that are primarily focused on better coordination and integration of health services before we turn to wider efforts to align health care, public health, and social services.

Patient-Centered Medical Home Model

First developed by the American Academy of Pediatrics in 1967, the patient-centered medical home (PCMH) model has gained significant traction in primary care in the last decade. The goal of this model is to provide "comprehensive, continuous, patient-centered, team-based, and accessible primary care in the context of a patient's family and community."[8] The Affordable Care Act promotes the implementation of the PCMH model in primary care and, with the growing adoption of value-based payment, many PCMH practices have become part of ACOs. Because PCMH is based on a recognition that health care should be provided with the whole person (and often whole family) in mind, the model has led the way in expanding the understanding of what types of professionals should be included in the health care team. In addition to a primary care physician, the PCMH team may include a registered nurse, a care manager, a social worker, a pharmacist, a behavioral health specialist, and, as we will describe in more detail later in the chapter, a lawyer.

By including multiple types of professionals under one roof, the PCMH improves access to and coordination of care as well as attention to the multiple factors that play a role in patient and population health. The PCMH is particularly useful in addressing the complex needs of vulnerable populations: "Providing patients with insurance coverage and a medical home has been found to reduce racial and ethnic disparities in access and quality of preventive and chronic care and to improve outcomes for vulnerable patient populations."[9] PCMHs are generally accessibly placed in the community and offer flexible hours to facilitate access to care. Many PCMH programs colocate with behavioral health and social service organizations (such as food banks), further supporting access to basic needs for vulnerable populations. While the PCMH model has been promoted by the ACA and by the medical community, it requires an infusion of resources to fully take hold. While payment reform has been helpful in shifting funding priorities away from a single focus on medical services to a broader array of services required to keep people healthy, the health care system still has a long way to go in making adequate investments to improve population health and reduce disparities.

Behavioral Health Integration into Primary Care

Another important health care system reform is the movement toward behavioral health services integration (BHI) into primary care. The term *behavioral health* "encompasses behavioral factors in chronic illness care, care of physical symptoms associated with stress rather than diseases, and health behaviors, as well as mental health and substance abuse conditions and diagnoses."[10] As discussed in the chapter on health disparities, there is a tremendous need for behavioral health services, particularly among vulnerable populations. People with mental health and substance use disorders have significantly worse physical health outcomes than those who do not suffer from these disorders. In fact, adults with serious mental illness die, on average, 25 years earlier than the general population,[11] and the recent opioid crisis has demonstrated the increased mortality rate for people with substance use disorders. People with mental health and substance use disorders are also more likely to engage in unhealthy behaviors such as smoking and eating a poor diet, making them more susceptible to chronic disease. Yet, access to primary care is often hampered by stigma, anxiety, or a chaotic life associated with mental illness or substance abuse.[12]

At the same time, many patients who *do* access primary care often find it difficult to navigate and access mental health and substance abuse services, such that their mental health needs may go undetected and unaddressed. **FIGURE 6.1** shows that people have difficulty accessing mental health services for a variety of reasons: cost, problems with insurance coverage, stigma, and lack of knowledge about how to access services. Despite the ACA's requirement that there be parity between insurance coverage for mental health services and primary care, there are still significant barriers to accessing the former. A recent study showed that many mental health providers do not participate in provider networks through the ACA insurance marketplaces, making those providers unaffordable for most consumers.[13] In 2012, the American Academy of Child and Adolescent Psychiatry estimated that only 15% to 25% of children with

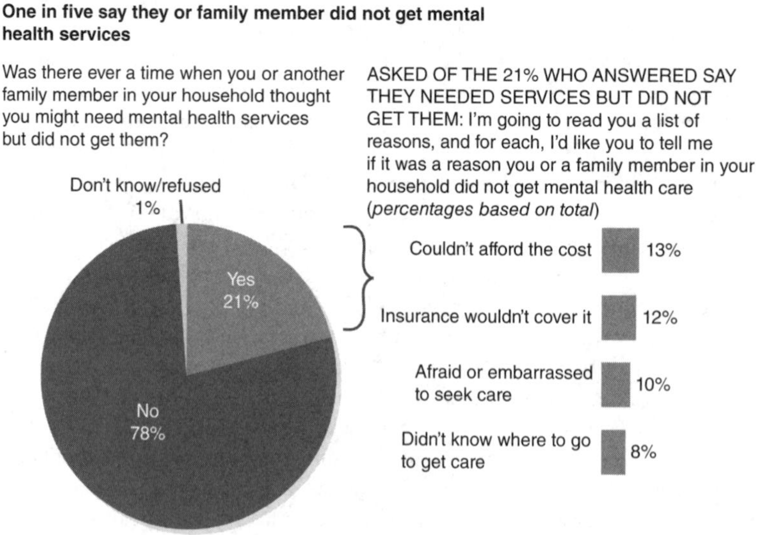

One in five say they or family member did not get mental health services

Was there ever a time when you or another family member in your household thought you might need mental health services but did not get them?

ASKED OF THE 21% WHO ANSWERED SAY THEY NEEDED SERVICES BUT DID NOT GET THEM: I'm going to read you a list of reasons, and for each, I'd like you to tell me if it was a reason you or a family member in your household did not get mental health care (*percentages based on total*)

Don't know/refused 1%

Yes 21%

No 78%

Couldn't afford the cost — 13%

Insurance wouldn't cover it — 12%

Afraid or embarrassed to seek care — 10%

Didn't know where to go to get care — 8%

FIGURE 6.1 One in five say they or family member did not get mental health services.

The Henry J. Kaiser Family Foundation, Kaiser Health Tracking Poll. April 2016. https://www.kff.org/.

psychiatric disorders received specialty care.[14] Consequently, diagnosis and management of behavioral health problems have generally fallen to primary care providers.

Until recently, the mental health and substance abuse care delivery systems have been largely separated from the health care system, leading to fragmented care (when mental health care is accessed at all), lack of coordinated management of physical and mental health problems, and significant access barriers. Along with other efforts to better coordinate care that is patient centered, BHI has been promoted as a way to integrate physical and behavioral health care. BHI has been described as "the approach and model of delivering care that comprehensively addresses the primary care, behavioral health, specialty care, and social support needs [of patients] with behavioral health issues in a manner that is continuous and family-centered."[15] You may detect a similarity in language between that describing BHI and the PCMH—comprehensive, continuous care that is patient and family centered. BHI, like the PCMH, is an effort to not only better coordinate care, but also to make care more accessible and responsive to patient needs, particularly for those from the most vulnerable populations.

Models of BHI vary according to the level of integration. At one end of the spectrum are efforts to simply better detect behavioral health needs through screening and to coordinate primary care and behavioral health services through referrals and follow-up. This approach creates a system for helping patients and families to navigate existing services and to facilitate better communication among providers. At the other end of the spectrum is full integration, in which behavioral health staff are fully integrated into the primary care practice (often a PCMH), working as a member of the health care team and providing direct services to patients. In the middle are models in which behavioral health services are colocated with primary care (e.g., located next door to the primary practice) in which providers refer back and forth and share patients, but the practices remain separate entities. **FIGURE 6.2** shows these different levels of integration.

One of the challenges to achieving full system integration is determining how services will be paid for. Traditional fee for service arrangements have caused considerable barriers to BHI by limiting reimbursement for the services that make BHI possible—consultations with specialists, care coordination, and services provided in one office on the same day (e.g., co-occurring visits with a primary care provider and a behavioral health specialist). However, value-based payment reforms are

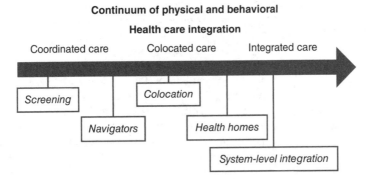

FIGURE 6.2 Continuum of physical and behavioral health care integration.

Kaiser Family Foundation. Integrating physical and behavioral health care: promising medicaid models, issue brief, executive summary. February 2014:3.

helping to facilitate BHI by allowing providers to bill for behavioral health services as part of primary care. (We describe later in this chapter other health care payment innovations that support payment for nonmedical and behavioral health services.)

Initial research indicates that BHI does improve outcomes. Specifically, studies of collaborative care management (in which "care or case managers systematically link patients with mental health and primary care providers") have found that this approach "improves mental health outcomes for patients with chronic medical conditions (e.g., chronic pain, diabetes, cardiovascular risk) and may improve medical outcomes, especially if care managers also address the medical conditions."[16] For the most vulnerable populations who struggle to access behavioral health services, BHI is a promising approach. However, policymakers have not yet fully embraced BHI by providing adequate infrastructure and funding to support systematic BHI across primary care providers.

Outreach to Connect the Clinic to the Community

One thing that a stronger focus on SDOH has made clear is that access to appropriate health care for vulnerable populations cannot be achieved simply by providing people with health insurance and building a clinic in the community. Given the substantial barriers to health and health care that vulnerable populations face, including a whole host of social factors, community health centers and other clinics are investing in ways to better connect clinical services to the community.

Community Health Workers and Community Health Teams

One of these investments has been in community health workers (CHWs). The American Public Health Association describes the role of the CHW this way: "A frontline public health worker who is a trusted member of and/or has an unusually close understanding of the community. This trusting relationship enables the worker to serve as a liaison/link/intermediary between health/social services and the community to facilitate access to services and improve the quality and cultural competence of service delivery."[17] CHWs help patients navigate the health care system, but may also make home visits to patients to support medication adherence or to counsel patients about preventive care. Increasingly, CHWs are trained to identify and address SDOH such as housing or neighborhood conditions affecting health and may engage in community organizing to support population health.

Another important approach to connecting the clinic to the community with a focus on addressing SDOH is the community health team (CHC). The ACA promotes community health teams as extensions of primary care, particularly as a way to support the PCMH model. The ACA describes the CHC as an interprofessional health care team that "may include medical specialists, nurses, pharmacists, nutritionists, dieticians, social workers, behavioral and mental health providers (substance use disorder prevention and treatment providers), doctors of chiropractic, licensed complementary and alternative medicine practitioners, and physicians' assistants."[18]

CHC members work with local primary care providers as well as community-based organizations and resources to coordinate care with a focus on chronic disease management. The goal of these teams is to "develop and implement care models that integrate clinical and community health promotion and preventive services for patients. Priority is given to patients with chronic diseases."[19] Given the increased prevalence of chronic disease among vulnerable populations and the clear linkages between SDOH and chronic disease, the interdisciplinary CHC approach may prove helpful in not only promoting access to higher quality health care for vulnerable populations, but also in identifying and addressing SDOH that stand in the way of health improvement. As with CHWs, investment in CHCs has been sporadic. Some states have invested Medicaid funding in CHCs. While research is limited as to the effect of community health teams on patient outcomes, some studies indicate that CHCs can help to improve the quality of care provided to patients as well as reduce costs.[20]

Clinical Approaches to Serving Specific Vulnerable Populations

A final health care delivery innovation worth describing is the growth of specialized clinics and clinical approaches that are tailored to specific populations based on their discrete needs. We highlight some of these efforts below.

Homeless Patients

With greater attention to and understanding of the complex health and social needs of the homeless population, a number of specialized clinics have been developed in recent years to meet these needs. In particular, the federal Veteran's Administration medical centers have created Homeless Patient-Aligned Care Teams (H-PACTs). The H-PACT is a multidisciplinary team (made up of physicians, nurses, social workers, behavioral health specialists, and substance abuse counselors) that not only provide medical services but also social supports, such as food, clothing, and assistance with finding safe stable housing, to homeless veterans.[21]

LGBT Patients

To address the specific needs of lesbian, gay, bisexual, and transgendered (LGBT) patients, a number of communities have developed specialized clinics, often within community health centers, in which providers are specially trained in LGBT health issues. Often these clinics are multidisciplinary, offering health services in coordination with other social services, and sometimes community advocacy as well. For example, the Los Angeles LGBT Center provides medical services, social services and housing, education, and advocacy, all under one roof.[22]

Children and Youth

While school-based health centers (SBHCs) are not new (they have been around for 40 years), they have "evolved from various public health needs to the development of a specific collaborative model of care that is sensitive to the unique needs of children and youth, as well as to vulnerable populations facing significant barriers to access."[23] SBHCs provide onsite care to children and youth through an interdisciplinary team of providers, including primary care and mental health providers who deliver immunizations, provide reproductive health services, and manage chronic illnesses such as obesity, asthma, and mental health disorders. Research shows that SBHCs not only improve access to care for vulnerable children and youth, they also improve health and educational outcomes.[24]

Patients Who Have Experienced Trauma

In the chapter on social and structural barriers to health, we described in some detail the roles that adverse childhood experiences (ACEs), toxic stress, and exposure to violence play in health. The relatively new understanding of the prevalence of trauma and its effects on both child and adult health has led to a clinical approach known as "trauma-informed care." Trauma can be caused by a single event, a series of events, or persistent exposure to traumatic conditions:

> Events or experiences that are traumatic for human beings include catastrophic environmental conditions (both natural and human influenced); various types of accidents; large-scale violence (e.g., war, genocide, torture, human trafficking, terrorism, and forced migration); "structural violence" that involves systematic oppression or discrimination (e.g., racism, homophobia, transphobia); interpersonal violence, family violence, childhood or adult sexual assault, abuse and neglect .... and life events that reduce trust or a sense of safety and security...[25]

The U.S. Substance Abuse and Mental Health Services Administration (SAMHSA) states that "a program, organization, or system that is trauma-informed:

1. *Realizes* the widespread impact of trauma and understands potential paths for recovery.
2. *Recognizes* the signs and symptoms of trauma in clients, families, staff, and others involved with the system.
3. *Responds* by fully integrating knowledge about trauma into policies, procedures, and practices.
4. Seeks to actively resist *re-traumatization*."[26]

SAMHSA also promotes six key principles in trauma-informed care: (1) safety; (2) trustworthiness and transparency; (3) peer support; (4) collaboration and mutuality; (5) empowerment, voice, and choice; and (6) cultural, historical, and gender issues.[27] Trauma-informed care may be particularly important for particular populations—such as veterans, victims of intimate partner violence (IPV), children living in poverty and/or experiencing abuse and neglect, and refugees from war-torn countries—likely to have experienced or who are still experiencing trauma.

The recent attention to ACEs has driven a growth in proposed policies that promote trauma-informed care. In March 2017, the National Conference of State Legislatures noted that there were 38 bills in 18 states that "included appropriating funds for ACEs prevention, establishing task forces or study committees, and requiring or encouraging health care providers to use an ACE screening tool with their patients."[28] Screening for IPV has also been promoted through policy. The Joint Commission on Accreditation of Health Care (JCAHO), an independent organization that accredits and certifies health care organizations and programs, and the Affordable Care Act both require screening for IPV in primary care. The Academy of Pediatrics has created screening tools for pediatric primary care providers to identify ACEs and toxic stress.[29] There are also a number of primary prevention programs that focus on preventing child abuse and neglect and on strengthening vulnerable families, such as home visiting programs. Ultimately, prevention of trauma is key to health equity: "Violence prevention, poverty elimination, education promotion, hunger prevention, homelessness prevention, and other strategies that eliminate social disparities all contribute to the prevention of life-altering trauma and the achievement of health equity."[30]

Despite exciting initiatives in health care to integrate population health principles, respond more effectively to SDOH, and address the particular needs of vulnerable populations, there are major gaps in the fight against health disparities. First, many of these efforts struggle with sustainable funding and policy support, which are subject to changing political winds. For example, many of these initiatives have been driven by directives and funding from the ACA, a law that is currently being (openly) undermined by the Trump Administration. Second, while these clinical innovations are an important step forward in promoting health equity, they still represent downstream approaches to the problem of health injustice. Clinical interventions, no matter how carefully designed to respond to chronic illness or the special needs of particular patient populations, alone cannot combat the upstream social ills that lead to poor population health and health inequity in the first place. In the next section, we move slightly further upstream to analyze efforts to better align clinical care, public health, and social services as a way to more systematically address SDOH and the root causes of health inequity.

▶ Aligning Health Care, Public Health, and Social Services

Recognition by health care system stakeholders that social factors are critical to health has led them to forge new partnerships with the public health sector. These partnerships hold a great deal of promise, as the two sectors have historically acted mostly independently of one another. A report by the Institute of Medicine in 2012, *Primary Care and Public Health: Exploring Integration to Improve Population Health*, pressed a new agenda—breaking down the silos between primary care and public health to facilitate shared goals and integration:

> Primary care and public health are uniquely positioned to play critical roles in tackling the complex health problems that exist both nationally and locally. They share a similar goal of health improvement and can build on this shared platform to catalyze intersectoral partnerships designed to bring about sustained improvements in population health.[31]

The attention to population health and SDOH in clinical care that we described above has encouraged health care systems and providers to seek new partnerships with their local public health departments, as well as with a range of community-based services and resources. The need for these partnerships has been made clear by the demands placed on physicians to address social needs as part of health care, and by the fact that most health care providers serving vulnerable populations do not feel equipped to respond to the multitude of their patients' social needs. A 2012 survey of physicians by the Robert Wood Johnson Foundation found that four out of five physicians said that "patients' social needs are as important to address as their medical conditions," and an equal number said they "do not feel confident in their capacity to meet their patients' social needs, and they believe this impedes their ability to provide quality care."[32] Some of the clinical programs and initiatives described above have helped support physicians to better respond to patients' social needs. But without ensuring that patients actually receive appropriate social services and access other community resources, it is difficult for health care providers to have much of an impact on SDOH.

While most agree that effective partnerships and alignments among health care, public health, and social services are critical to addressing SDOH and health disparities, connecting these traditionally siloed systems is challenging. It also begs some important questions. What role does each sector play? Who takes the lead in identifying social needs and who is responsible for addressing them? What systems and infrastructure are required to sustain healthy, effective partnerships that keep patient and population health at the center? In this section, we explore these questions by analyzing some of the existing efforts to build partnerships focused on addressing patients' social needs in alignment with health care. Here, we introduce a new term that is now being used to describe social needs that impact health: *health-related social needs* (HRSN). Specifically, we consider: (1) screening: who is responsible for screening patients for HRSNs and what happens to the information collected? (2) data: how are data from individual electronic health records, health insurance claims databases, and public health surveillance systems being used to guide SDOH interventions? and (3) financing: what are some of the health care financing mechanisms that are being explored to address HRSNs in a more systematic and upstream way?

Screening for Health-Related Social Needs

As we have highlighted elsewhere, the U.S. is exceptional among peer nations in its mismatch between funding for health care and social services. Because safety net programs, such as subsidized housing, income supports, and health insurance, are limited and do not meet the need, connecting people to adequate supports can be challenging. But even prior to helping people to access supports and services, their specific needs must first be identified. Many low-income and vulnerable people are not aware of what resources are available to them or that they have rights under the law that may help them access those resources. Like the health care system, social service (and legal-aid) systems are generally fragmented and difficult to navigate. In most communities, there is not a single location or agency where a person or family can go to assess their needs and connect them to resources. With health care's focus on SDOH (and on reducing health care costs associated with SDOH-driven chronic illnesses), screening for HRSNs is becoming more common as part of primary care.

While taking a patient's social history (such as asking about a patient's smoking habits, alcohol use, and sexual behavior) has long been part of the traditional medical interview in primary care, including questions about socioeconomic factors that may affect health, such as poverty, substandard housing, and food insecurity, is a relatively recent phenomenon. There is no one validated tool that providers use to screen for social conditions and basic needs affecting health, but in recent years there has been a proliferation of tools, and some health systems are working to integrate social needs screening questions into their electronic medical records. One example that has been in existence for more than a decade is the IHELLP tool, which was developed for the pediatric field and asks questions about income, housing, education, literacy, legal status, and personal safety. See **TABLE 6.1**.

The integration of screening for HRSNs into primary care begs a few questions. Who should be responsible for administering the screening? Primary care

TABLE 6.1 Examples of Potential Social History Questions (Using the "IHELLP" Mnemonic) to Address Basic Needs

Domain/Area	Examples of Questions
Income	
General	Do you ever have trouble making ends meet?
Food income	Do you ever have a time when you don't have enough food? Do you have WIC? Food stamps?
Housing	
Housing	Is your housing ever a problem for you?
Utilities	Do you ever have trouble paying your electric/heat/telephone bill?
Education	
Appropriate education placement	How is your child doing in school? Is he/she getting the help to learn what he/she needs?
Early childhood program	Is your child in Head Start, preschool, or other early childhood enrichment?
Legal status	
Immigration	Do you have questions about your immigration status? Do you need help accessing benefits or services for your family?
Literacy	
Child literacy	Do you read to your child every night?
Parent literacy	How happy are you with how you read?
Personal safety	
Domestic violence	Have you ever taken out a restraining order? Do you feel safe in your relationship?
General safety	Do you feel safe in your home? In your neighborhood?

Kenyon C, Sandel M, Silverstein M, et al. Revisiting the social history for child health. *Pediatrics*. September 2007;120(3): e734–e738.

physicians have limited time with patients (often as little as 15 minutes). Some stakeholders suggest that it is not reasonable to add a social needs screening to an already harried and full agenda for the primary care visit. The advent of the health care team has helped to alleviate this problem by providing opportunity for screening to be completed by other health care professionals, including physician assistants, care managers, community health workers, or others. This way, information from the screening can be shared with the primary care physician or nurse who can incorporate it into a treatment plan. But it can also be shared with a social worker or case manager, who can help to connect patients and families with resources.

The second question that often arises when HRSN screening is integrated into health care is: what if the health care team is unable to respond to the need identified? This is a common problem for primary care providers, as many do not work with onsite social workers or other professionals whose job it is to follow up on these types of issues. Providers may feel overwhelmed by the level of need of their patients, as well as ill-equipped to direct patients to appropriate resources or to follow up to see if they have actually accessed those resources. To address this problem, a number of web-based searchable database platforms have been developed to help clinicians identify appropriate community resources for patients. These databases support the ability of providers to connect individual patients to community resources and help to develop partnerships between health care and social service agencies. But, as helpful as these partnerships are, they do not create the kind of systems change that is required to significantly impact population health disparities. Increasingly, health care systems, in partnership with public health agencies and other community partners, are using data to target interventions toward the most vulnerable patients populations and to identify specific community conditions that must be altered to improve population health.

Data-Driven Strategies

One thing that the health care and public health systems have an abundance of is data. The electronic medical record, in which each patient's health history and medical care are recorded and updated each time he or she interacts with the health care system, has become a valuable source of information—not just for the patient and provider, but also for tracking individual and population-level outcomes. Another source of data that is helpful to understanding population health, including health disparities, are insurance claims databases, which can help to identify high-need, high-risk patients whose complex social needs may drive overutilization of medical care. And finally, long an important resource for public health surveillance of disease trends, public health data are increasingly being used to better track health disparities. Below we describe some of the ways that different types of data are being utilized to inform interventions both within the health care system and outside of it. Furthermore, you will notice that some of these efforts explicitly connect different types of data to understand the role of social determinants in health outcomes and to inform community-based interventions.

Hotspotting

While providing care to some of the poorest and most vulnerable patients in Camden, New Jersey, family physician Jeffrey Brenner had an idea. Frustrated by not being able to better address the needs of highly vulnerable and complex patients, he created a searchable database using claims and hospital discharge data from all patients at Camden's hospitals, mapping them geographically. He found that a very small number of patients were driving a disproportionate share of health care costs. Using this approach, now known as "hotspotting," Brenner used the data to identify and direct resources to the most high-risk patients. In 2002, he created the Camden Coalition, which builds collaborations among community-based primary care providers, frontline hospital staff and social workers, and other community partners from across Camden to provide a team-based approach to managing medical care and social needs of complex patients. The teams receive daily information about hospitalizations, which helps them track complex patients and identify when interventions are needed. The model is based on building trust and long-term relationships with patients and their families.[33] Brenner's hotspotting model has been replicated in many locations across the country. In 2017, the National Center for Complex Health and Social Needs was launched to inform and support data-driven and patient-centered approaches to patients with complex needs through collaborations among clinicians, social service partners, policymakers, researchers, and consumers.[34]

Geomarkers

While Dr. Brenner used data to target interventions toward complex patients, others are linking clinical data with community-level data to identify particular health risks. Dr. Andrew Beck and colleagues coined the term "geomarkers" (like biomarkers used to predict disease) to demonstrate place-based (i.e., neighborhood-level) risk factors for poor health outcomes. Beck and colleagues define "geomarkers" as "'any objective, contextual, or geographic measure' that influences or predicts the incidence of outcome or disease. By complementing biology with geography, we are able to tap into health-relevant data that generally exist in isolation from clinical care."[35] Geomarkers can include a range of neighborhood factors known to affect health—e.g., the poverty rate, housing code violations, and accessibility of health care. **TABLE 6.2** shows community-level geomarkers and potential interventions.

Linking community-based data with health data provides the opportunity to better understand individual susceptibility based on community status and to guide public health interventions and public health partnerships. But it can also help clinicians to better manage population health and identify social factors driving disparities. Beck and colleagues argue:

> If used effectively, these data could simulate a visit to a patient's home community, informing care in real time. They could "take the pulse" of communities of interest, identifying the acuity (and distribution) of risk to warn providers of need for action. Just as abnormal laboratory tests or vital signs warn of a patient's potential for clinical deterioration, so too may place-based "community vital signs" warn of social determinants of health–related concerns.[36]

Using data to inform clinical, public health, and community-based interventions is an effective way to target limited resources and inform clinical and population health strategies, particularly with regard to vulnerable populations. But databases are not the only way to gather and use data to address community health needs. Gathering information and data from patients and community members is

TABLE 6.2 Community-Level Geomarkers

Community-level geomarkers specific to the health service, physical, economic, and psychosocial environments and potential Interventions that could be relevant at the population or patient level

Health service environment	Physical environment	Economic environment	Psychosocial environment
GEOMARKERS			
Distance to pharmacy Live within "pharmacy desert" Pharmacy quality metric Distance to primary care Live within undeserved area Vehicle availability Public transport availability	Housing code violations Vacancy rate Renter rate Home value Crowding/ population density Exposure to pollution	Poverty rate Household income Home ownership Car ownership Educational attainment	Crime rate Mental health access
INTERVENTIONS			
Medication delivery Care coordination Community health worker Home nurse visitation Medicaid rides Telemedicine	Housing inspection Legal advocacy Air conditioning or filtration Development of affordable housing	Financial services Medicaid rides Legal advocacy Public benefit procurement Community health worker Community agency referrals	Community health worker Community agency referrals Resilience training Community partnerships

Beck AF, Sandel MT, Ryan PH, et al. Mapping neighborhood health geomarkers to clinical care decisions to promote equity in child health. *Health Affairs.* June 1, 2017;36(6):999–1005.

also critical to informing health system change and reallocation of resources toward addressing HRSNs.

Community Health Needs Assessments

Our first two examples of data-driven population health initiatives have involved clinicians who have identified the need for stronger partnerships among health care, public health, and community partners to effectively address SDOH. In general, hospitals have not traditionally actively sought ways to engage with community partners around SDOH. To put it bluntly, hospitals have not had much incentive to focus on primary prevention since their revenue comes from people needing medical care and from keeping their hospital beds full. The Affordable Care Act has helped move hospitals more squarely into the conversation about the community factors that drive poor health outcomes. The law requires that, in order to maintain their tax-exempt status, not-for-profit hospitals must conduct a community health needs assessment (CHNA) at least every three years. These needs assessments must include input from the community, including the local public health department as well as from medically underserved, low-income and minority communities. Hospitals must also devise an implementation strategy to address the community health needs identified in the CHNA. **FIGURE 6.3** shows an example of the types of data collection used in a CHNA and how that data is used to identify and prioritize the health needs that should be addressed in the implementation strategy and monitored over time.

Under what is known as the "community benefit" standard, the federal Internal Revenue Service (IRS) has long required that a not-for-profit hospital demonstrate that it is contributing to the community in exchange for a tax exemption. Prior to the ACA, most community benefit spending took the form of reimbursing the hospital for charity care—providing care to the uninsured or making up for the gap between the cost of treating Medicaid patients and the amount reimbursed by the government—but not for community-based activities focused on health improvement.[37] The ACA's new CHNA mandate was an attempt to refocus not-for-profit hospitals on upstream population health efforts through engagement with their

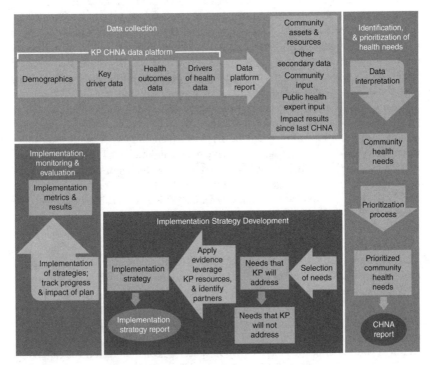

FIGURE 6.3 Community health needs assessment process.

Courtesy of Kaiser Permanente.

local communities. The IRS regulations supporting the ACA mandate are explicit that CHNAs must pay attention to SDOH by defining health needs as "not only the need to address financial and other barriers to care but also the need to prevent illness, to ensure adequate nutrition, or to address social, behavioral, and environmental factors that influence health in the community."[38]

The CHNA has opened up an avenue for communication and collaboration between health care, public health, and the community to identify and address community-level factors that contribute to disease and perpetuate health disparities. But asking hospitals to invest in community health is a cultural shift. As Lawrence Massa, President of the Minnesota Hospital Association, told *The Washington Post*: "Caring for the health of people before they come into the hospital is unfamiliar territory. Not everyone took naturally to it. We saw some communities that embraced this and did a nice job. ... In other communities, there's been friction between public health and the acute setting—and lack of understanding."[39] Breaking down the silos between health care, public health, and the community takes a concerted effort. The ACA's CHNA mandate is an important step in beginning to form those partnerships. Yet, with uncertainty around the future of the ACA, it is hard to predict how sustainable these budding relationships will be.

Financing Social Service Integration to Improve Health

The mismatch between funding for health care and social services in the U.S. has led researchers and policymakers to assess the potential value of shifting resources toward better integration of health and social services, both in terms of improving the health of vulnerable populations and reducing health care costs. A study by the Blue Cross Blue Shield of Massachusetts Foundation evaluated the evidence regarding whether increased investment in social services and partnerships between health care and social services influences health outcomes and health care costs. They found that selected social services—specifically housing support for low-income individuals and families, nutritional assistance for high-risk women, infants and children, and older adults, and case management and community outreach for high-need low-income families, older adults, and children with asthma—all demonstrated health care cost savings and better health outcomes for those receiving services. Furthermore, the study found that income supports such as the earned income tax credit and Social Security disability income are associated with better health outcomes. Providing high-quality early childhood education to children ages zero to five from disadvantaged backgrounds is also correlated with improved adult health outcomes.[40] This evidence, combined with the trend toward value-based payment for health care, has encouraged policymakers and health systems to consider investment in social service integration.[41]

One important federal investment has been the Center for Medicare and Medicaid Innovation's (CMMI) Accountable Health Communities (AHC) grant program. CMMI describes the AHC as addressing "a critical gap between clinical care and community services in the current health care delivery system by testing whether systematically identifying and addressing the health-related social needs of Medicare and Medicaid beneficiaries' through screening, referral, and community navigation services will impact health care costs and reduce health care utilization."[42] Grantees will test effective health care-social service collaboration through a community bridge organization that will link patients and community members to the services they need. **FIGURE 6.4** demonstrates how this model is intended to work.

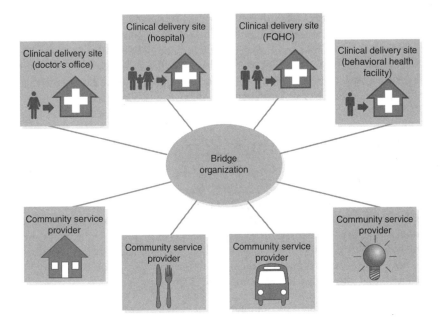

FIGURE 6.4 Accountable health community.

Courtesy of Centers for Medicare and Medicaid Services (CMS) – visit www.cms.gov.

At the state level, policymakers are also experimenting with state investments in social service integration, particularly through their Medicaid programs. Under federal law, states may apply for a waiver (called a Section 1115 waiver based on the Social Security Act provision from which it comes) from federal Medicaid program requirements to test and evaluate program innovations. One way states have used these waivers is to expand services not typically offered through the Medicaid program. The waiver is only granted if these services can be shown to be budget neutral and have potential to reduce costs and improve care. A number of states—including Oregon, Texas, New York, and Vermont—are using Section 1115 waivers to pay for a range of nonmedical services to improve patient care and outcomes.[43] One promising development is state efforts to fund supportive housing to Medicaid beneficiaries. For example, through its 1115 waiver, Oregon created regional coordinated care organizations that have the authority to fund housing improvements, temporary housing after hospital stays, and moving expenses if they can be shown to be health related.[44] Some suggest that Medicaid funds be made available to pay directly for supportive housing (e.g., rent) for people with chronic medical or psychiatric illness as a way to reduce health care costs (e.g., hospitalizations and emergency room use) and prevent homelessness.[45] Others propose that hospitals should contribute to these costs.[46] States also have the option to fund case management services for patients under Sections 1905 and 1915 of the Medicaid law. This allows for the hiring of case managers who can assist beneficiaries in accessing social, educational, and other services.

Up to this point, we have focused primarily on innovations in the health care delivery system designed to better address HRSNs within the health care system and through public health and community partnerships. As promising as some of these efforts are in beginning to tackle persistent health disparities and improve health care for vulnerable populations, they do not fundamentally change the larger systemic and structural conditions that lead to poor health in the first place. In the next section, we move even further upstream to consider how law, policy, and larger-scale public health interventions can be used to improve the environments in which people live with an eye toward improving population health.

▶ Moving Upstream: Federal, State, and Local Initiatives

We have emphasized throughout this text that, discrete from access to or the quality of the health care system, societal structures (e.g., discrimination, inequality, a modest and difficult-to-access safety net, a hazardous environment) strongly influence the likely health trajectory of individuals and populations. These societal structures do not evolve naturally. They are the result of history, laws, policies, and funding decisions that ultimately shape the conditions in which people live:

> Laws transform the underpinnings of the health system and also act at various points in and on the complex environments that generate the conditions for health. Those environments include the widely varied policy context of multiple government agencies, such as education, energy, and transportation agencies, as well as many statutes, regulations, and court cases intended to reshape the factors that improve or impede health.[47]

In recent years, there has been growing recognition that to truly improve population health and reduce health disparities, systems and structural reforms outside of the health care system are as important as those within it. To accomplish real change, there needs to be a shift in focus away from interventions that affect individuals one at a time toward large-scale interventions. Many of these interventions require law and policy change. **FIGURE 6.5** demonstrates the potential impact of interventions to influence health (including laws and policies) across a spectrum, from individual encounters with providers to large-scale societal change.

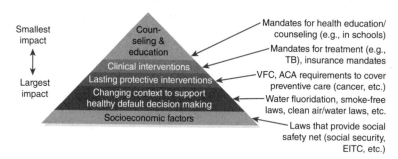

FIGURE 6.5 Health impact pyramid with legal intervention.

Modified from Frieden, TR. A framework for public health action: the health impact pyramid. *American Journal of Public Health*. April 2010;100(4):590–595.

Health in All Policies

This perspective on the role of law and policy in shaping the conditions that either support or harm health has led to calls for a "Health in All Policies" (HIAP) approach to policymaking. HIAP is "a collaborative approach to improving the health of all people by incorporating health considerations into decision-making across sectors and policy areas."[48] This approach has been promoted at the federal level through the Surgeon General's National Prevention Strategy[49] and has been adopted by some state governments, most notably in California. HIAP recognizes the multifactorial nature of health determinants:

> Health in All Policies is a response to a variety of complex and often inex-
> tricably linked problems such as the chronic illness epidemic, growing
> inequality and health inequities, rising health care costs, an aging popula-
> tion, climate change and related threats to our natural resources, and the
> lack of efficient strategies for achieving governmental goals with shrinking
> resources.[50]

Health Impact Assessments

A related effort is the health impact assessment (HIA), which is "a tool that can help communities, decision makers, and practitioners make choices that improve public health through community design." Specifically, "HIA brings potential positive and negative public health impacts and considerations to the decision-making process for plans, projects, and policies that fall outside traditional public health arenas, such as transportation and land use."[51]

At the local level, there are efforts to bring together the community devel-opment and health sectors to address issues such as access to health care and healthy food, early childhood education, and opportunities for physical activity and health promotion in schools, workplaces, and neighborhoods. Increasingly, banks and other financial institutions support these community development efforts.[52] In addition, state and local redevelopment agencies charged with planning and financing community improvement and economic development projects are considering population health in their designs. Specifically, these agencies are often tasked with addressing blight—which may be defined under state or local law as including "public health risks like unsafe or unhealthy buildings and the presence of hazardous waste"—as well as the "lack of access to services such as grocery stores and pharmacies."[53] Focusing community devel-opment and redevelopment efforts on population health is critical to address-ing SDOH and for leveling the playing field for people living in low-income neighborhoods.

Community Driven Efforts

While policy and planning are fundamental to improving the social condi-tions of people living in disadvantaged communities, top-down efforts that do not engage people in those communities are less likely to be successful. In the chapter on advocacy for health justice, we describe in more detail the role of

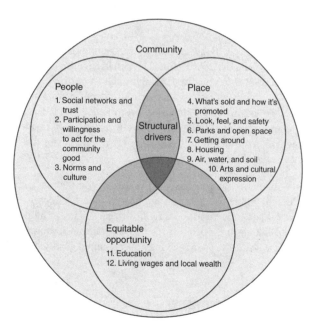

FIGURE 6.6 Tool for Health and Resilience In Vulnerable Environments.

Data from The Prevention Institute. Tool for Health and Resilience in Vulnerable Environments. https://www.preventioninstitute.org /tools/thrive-tool-health-resilience-vulnerable-environments.

community organizing and engagement in social change and community health. Here, we highlight one effort designed around engaging community members in prioritizing actions focused on improving health. An instrument called THRIVE (Tool for Health and Resilience In Vulnerable Environments), created by a not-for-profit organization in California named the Prevention Institute, is intended to help communities assess and act on the "community determinants of health." THRIVE is a "a framework for understanding how structural drivers, such as racism, play out at the community level in terms of the social-cultural, physical/built, and economic/educational environments."[54] **FIGURE 6.6** describes how the THRIVE tool assesses and helps communities to act on structural drivers of health.

▶ Linking Health, Law, and Justice

Throughout this text, we have described the multiple and complex pathways between structural and legal factors and health inequity. We have also outlined how low-income and vulnerable populations suffer from severely inadequate access to justice and from laws and policies that fail to address health-related social needs. Greater recognition of these legal and structural barriers to health equity has driven partnerships among legal advocates, health care, and social service providers to challenge systems that fail to meet the needs of (and harm) the health of vulnerable populations. One critical initiative in this regard is the medical-legal partnership (MLP), which embeds lawyers and other legal professionals in health care institutions (e.g., ACOs, hospitals, PCMHs, and community health centers) to address the legal and structural issues that impede health and reinforce health disparities. MLPs work upstream to address the needs of vulnerable patients and populations:

> Attorneys in general—and poverty lawyers in particular—have an in-depth understanding of relevant policies, laws, and systems, and seek out solutions at the individual and policy levels to a range of health-related social and legal needs. When embedded as specialists in a health care setting, lawyers can directly resolve specific problems for individual patients, while also helping clinical and non-clinical staff navigate system and policy barriers and transform institutional practices.[55]

MLPs address many of the HRSNs affecting the health of vulnerable populations that we have described in this text: access to safety net programs and education, housing quality and safety, employment issues, barriers to care for immigrants, and family and community violence. These partnerships, of which there are now some 300 in 41 states, focus on the specific needs of the populations they serve—from maternal health and early childhood to veterans and the elderly.[56] By collaborating with health care and social service partners, MLPs not only strengthen service provision to vulnerable populations, they also help to identify the upstream social, structural, and legal issues that contribute to health disparities. Through legal advocacy, MLPs challenge the unfair practices and lack of enforcement of existing laws that impact health, and also help to promote law and policy changes designed to better protect the health of vulnerable populations. Some studies suggest that MLPs have a positive effect on health outcomes, especially for those with chronic illnesses such as asthma and sickle cell anemia, and reduce health care utilization and costs for high-risk adults.[57] Finally, one of the key features of MLPs is their ability to bring together and train health care, public health, legal, and social service providers to understand HSRNs though a structural and legal lens.

▶ The Next Generation: Education for Change

The persistence of health inequity in the U.S. has led to efforts in health professions education to better train students to recognize and identify SDOH, work in interdisciplinary teams, build skills in patient and policy advocacy, and explore systemic solutions to entrenched disparities. These efforts aim to shift the focus of health professions education from acute medical conditions to the broader perspective of population health and prevention.[58] As described earlier in the chapter, many health system changes have also followed this path, such as the PCMH and ACO models of care. Recently, the American Medical Association has promoted the idea that "knowledge and skills limited to the scientific basis of diseases, diagnoses, and treatments"[59] learned through basic and clinical science is insufficient for the effective practice of medicine. They propose that medical educators should adopt a third science in addition to the basic and clinical sciences—"health systems science," through which "physicians in training and health professions students must understand the broader system of health care, principles of policy and economics, population health management, interprofessional collaboration, behavioral and social determinants of health, and health system improvement."[60]

At the same time, educators in law, public policy, and the social sciences are increasingly acknowledging the fundamental role that health inequity plays in reinforcing social inequality and disadvantage. This has led to interprofessional education initiatives that bring together health professions students with students from social work, law, public policy, and other disciplines, in order to teach students strategies for interprofessional problem-solving around complex HSRNs. Medical-legal partnerships (described above) have been at the forefront of this type of interdisciplinary education.[61]

Still, these types of educational innovations have not yet been institutionalized. Some argue that for education to truly affect health inequity, academic institutions (including those in medicine, nursing, dentistry, public health, social work, and law) need to teach and model a truly social mission:

> [T]he unqualified commitment of these institutions to teaching and modeling social mission is needed, as are the voices of academic professional organizations, accrediting bodies, and student groups who have important roles in defining the values of young professionals… The commitments needed are not the domain of any one profession, and collaborative initiatives at the educational level will reinforce social mission norms in practice.[62]

As health professions education adapts to the demands of an evolving health care system and the complex social factors driving population health, there has also been a strong emphasis on expanding the competencies that students must demonstrate to become professionals in their fields. Some of the competencies include the ability to identify SDOH, to work effectively as part of an interdisciplinary team, and to demonstrate "cultural competence" in working with diverse patient populations. But some have criticized the current approach to teaching about health inequity and the focus on these types as competencies for two reasons. First, this approach fails to fully address the underlying structural factors that influence health and perpetuate health inequity. Second, they do not provide future practitioners with concrete strategies for addressing structural factors:

> [M]ost SDOH approaches place far less emphasis on the fact that it is the *unequal distribution* of money, power, and resources at global, national, and local levels that results in health disparities… Importantly, there are two tacit assumptions behind such educational efforts: first, that the SDOH are somehow "natural"—that is, not due to human made societal systems of power and privilege that give rise to inequities but, rather, to immutable facts of nature. Second is the assumption that teaching about the SDOH will somehow result in action to alleviate these inequities.[63]

To combat the potential for students to believe that SDOH may be addressed through cultural competence (which focuses on the discrete issues of the individual patient), Jonathan Metzl and Helena Hansen have proposed that students be required to develop "structural competency." They explain that development of structural competency includes five core training components: "(1) recognizing the structures that shape clinical interactions, (2) developing an extra-clinical language of structure; (3) rearticulating "cultural" formulations in structural terms; (4) observing and imagining structural interventions; and (5) developing structural humility."[64] Structural competency is intended to give students the ability not only to identify structural factors in health inequity, but also strategies and tools to advocate for change. In the chapter on advocacy for health justice, we explore in more detail the ways in which health care providers and their partners can advocate for structural change.

Another educational approach recently deployed to address health inequity is teaching students to recognize, monitor, and manage their own implicit biases. As we discussed in the chapter on the effects of discrimination and implicit bias on health and health care, implicit biases are "biases, stereotypes, and associations that exist outside conscious awareness [that] may adversely influence the health of minority, underserved, and stigmatized populations."[65] Research demonstrates that health care provider biases can negatively affect patient care and treatment. For example, one study showed that "despite consciously expressing explicit egalitarian goals, physicians were less likely to recommend thrombolysis [medication to dissolve blood clots] to African American patients, as compared with Caucasians with similar symptoms."[66] Some educators emphasize that a few didactic sessions discussing the role of implicit bias in perpetuating health disparities is inadequate, but Sukhera and Watling propose six key features necessary for education about implicit bias: "(1) creating a safe and nonthreatening learning context; (2) increasing knowledge about the science of implicit bias; (3) emphasizing how implicit bias influences behaviors and patient outcomes; (4) increasing self-awareness of existing implicit biases; (5) improving conscious efforts to overcome implicit bias; and (6) enhancing awareness of how implicit bias influences others."[67] Although little research exists to date on the efficacy of implicit bias education, educators engaged in these efforts emphasize that sustained attention to the issue of implicit bias in health care is needed to move the needle on health inequity. Increasing the number of health care providers from demographic backgrounds that more closely mirror patient populations is also an important factor in improving the care of vulnerable populations.

▶ Conclusion

This chapter has highlighted the many efforts being undertaken in the health care and public health systems to better integrate health and social services and to promote health equity in communities. In addition, we described the growing recognition of the significance of structural, legal, and policy underpinnings in health inequity and some of the intersectoral collaborations such as medical-legal partnerships, health impact assessments, and Health in All Policies initiatives centered around upstream systems changes. Finally, we discussed how educational reforms are focusing on better ways to train the next generation of health care providers, social workers, lawyers, and others to work more upstream to address social and structural factors in health inequity.

As important as all of these initiatives are in moving the U.S. down the path toward health equity, they cannot, in and of themselves, eliminate health disparities. To effect the systemic changes needed to improve population health and promote health justice, federal policies and funding priorities will need to align with the evidence: that treating all people with dignity and supporting them to meet their basic needs is key to improving population health. Health care teams, public health professionals, and lawyers can help facilitate better coordination between health and social service and help individuals to access legal entitlements. But they cannot create resources that do not exist, such as affordable housing or health insurance for those who struggle to stay afloat. Indeed, large-scale policy advocacy, along with health system change and local and state innovations, are required to truly tackle health inequity. In the next chapter, we explore strategies for how professionals concerned about health justice can advocate for change both within and outside of the health care system.

References

1. Berwick DM, Nolan TW, Whittington J. The triple aim: care, health, and cost. *Health Affairs.* 2008;27(3):759–769.
2. Wilson N, George P, Huber JM. Population health. In: Skochelak SE, Hawkins RE, Lawson LE, et al., eds. *Health Systems Science.* Philadelphia, PA: Elsevier; 2017: 121–122.
3. Woolf SH, Aron LY. The US health disadvantage relative to other high-income countries: findings from a National Research Council/Institute of Medicine report. *JAMA.* 2013;309:771–772.
4. Bauer UE, Briss PA, Goodman RA, Bowman BA. Prevention of chronic disease in the 21st century: elimination of the leading preventable causes of premature death and disability in the USA. *Lancet.* July 2016;384:45–46.
5. Starr SR, Nesse RE. The health care delivery system. In: Skochelak SE, Hawkins RE, Lawson LE, et al., eds. *Health Systems Science.* Philadelphia, PA: Elsevier; 2017: 26.
6. Starr SR, Nesse RE. The health care delivery system. In Skochelak SE, Hawkins RE, Lawson LE, et al., eds. *Health Systems Science.* Philadelphia, PA: Elsevier; 2017: 32–33.
7. Gottlieb L, Manchanda R, Sandel M. Practical strategies in addressing social determinants of health. In: King TE, Wheeler MB, Fernandez A, et al., eds. *Medical Management of Vulnerable & Underserved Patients: Principles, Practice, and Populations.* 2nd ed. New York, NY: McGraw Hill Professional Publishing; 2016: 98.
8. Berenson RA, Hammons T, Gans DN, et al. A house is not home: keeping patients at the center of practice redesign. *Health Affairs.* 2008;27(5):1219–1230.
9. Gupta R, Bodenheimer T. Creating the medical home for underserved patients. In: King TE, Wheeler MB, Fernandez A, et al., eds. *Medical Management of Vulnerable & Underserved Patients: Principles, Practice, and Populations.* 2nd ed. New York, NY: McGraw Hill Professional Publishing; 2016: 116.
10. Agency for Healthcare Research and Quality. What is integrated behavioral health care (IBHC)? Available at: https://integrationacademy.ahrq.gov/resources/ibhc-measures-atlas /what-integrated-behavioral-health-care-ibhc. Accessed January 11, 2018.
11. The Henry J. Kaiser Family Foundation. Integrating physical and behavioral health care: promising Medicaid models. *Issue Brief;* February 2014:1. Available at: https://www.kff.org /medicaid/issue-brief/integrating-physical-and-behavioral-health-care-promising-medicaid -models/. Accessed January 11, 2018.
12. Gerrity M. Evolving models of behavioral health integration: evidence update 2010–2015. Milbank Memorial Fund Report; May 2016. Available at: https://www.milbank.org /publications/evolving-models-of-behavioral-health-integration-evidence-update-2010-2015/. Accessed January 11, 2018.
13. Zhu JM, Zhang Y, Polsky D. Networks in ACA marketplaces are narrower for mental health care than for primary care. *Health Affairs.* 2017;36(9):1624–1631.

14. American Academy of Child and Adolescent Psychiatry Committee on Health Care Access and Economics Task Force on Mental Health. Improving mental health services in primary care: reducing administrative and financial barriers to access and collaboration. *Pediatrics.* 2009;123(4):1248–1251.

15. U.S. Substance Abuse and Mental Health Services Administration, U.S. Department of Health and Human Services Health Resources and Services Administration (SAMHSA-HRSA) Center for Integrated Health Solutions (CIHS). Integrating behavioral health and primary care for children and youth. Available at: http://www.integration.samhsa.gov/integrat- ed-care -models/13_June_CIHS_Integrated_Care_System_for_Children_final.pdf.

16. Gerrity M. Evolving models of behavioral health integration: evidence update 2010–2015. Milbank Memorial Fund Report; May 2016: 4. Available at: https://www.milbank .org/publications/evolving-models-of-behavioral-health-integration-evidence-update -2010–2015/.

17. American Public Health Association. Community health workers. Available at: https:// www.apha.org/apha-communities/member-sections/community-health-workers. Accessed January 11, 2018.

18. *The Patient Protection and Affordable Care Act.* §42 U.S.C. 18031 (2010); §3502(4).

19. The Association of State and Territorial Health Officials. Community health teams (issue report). Available at: http://www.astho.org/Programs/Access/Primary-Care/_Materials /Community-Health-Teams-Issue-Report/.

20. Takach M, Buxbaum J. Care management for Medicaid enrollees through community health teams. The Commonwealth Fund; May 2013. Available at: http://www.commonwealthfund .org/publications/fund-reports/2013/may/care-management.

21. Wilson N, George P, Huber JM. Population health. In: Skochelak SE, Hawkins RE, Lawson LE, et al., eds. *Health Systems Science.* Philadelphia, PA: Elsevier; 2017: 128.

22. Los Angeles LGBT Center website. Available at: https://lalgbtcenter.org/. Accessed January 11, 2018.

23. Keeton V, Soleimanpour S, Brindis CD. School-based health centers in an era of health care reform: building on history. *Current Problems in Pediatric and Adolescent Health Care.* July 2012;42(6):132–158.

24. Keeton V, Soleimanpour S, Brindis CD. School-based health centers in an era of health care reform: building on history. *Current Problems in Pediatric and Adolescent Health Care.* July 2012;42(6):132–158.

25. Kimberg L. Trauma and trauma-informed care. In: King TE, Wheeler MB, Fernandez A, et al., eds. *Medical Management of Vulnerable & Underserved Patients: Principles, Practice, and Populations.* 2nd ed. New York, NY: McGraw Hill Professional Publishing; 2016: 408.

26. Substance Abuse and Mental Health Services Administration (SAMHSA). Trauma-informed approach and trauma-specific interventions. Available at: https://www.samhsa.gov/nctic /trauma-interventions. Accessed January 11, 2018.

27. Substance Abuse and Mental Health Services Administration (SAMHSA). Trauma-informed approach and trauma-specific interventions. Available at: https://www.samhsa.gov/nctic /trauma-interventions. Accessed January 11, 2018.

28. National Conference of State Legislatures. State strategies for preventing child and adolescent injuries and violence health; August 2017. Available at: http://www.ncsl.org/documents /health/PreventingInjury2017.pdf.

29. American Academy of Pediatrics. Clinical assessment tools. Available at: https://www.aap .org/en-us/advocacy-and-policy/aap-health-initiatives/resilience/Pages/Clinical-Assessment -Tools.aspx.

30. Kimberg L. Trauma and trauma-informed care. In: King TE, Wheeler MB, Fernandez A, et al., eds. *Medical Management of Vulnerable & Underserved Patients: Principles, Practice, and Populations.* 2nd ed. New York, NY: McGraw Hill Professional Publishing; 2016: 419.

31. Institute of Medicine. Primary care and public health: exploring integration to improve population health; 2012: 17. Available at: http://www.nationalacademies.org/hmd /Reports/2012/Primary-Care-and-Public-Health.aspx.

32. Robert Wood Johnson Foundation. Health care's blind side. Available at: https://www.rwjf .org/en/library/research/2011/12/health-care-s-blind-side.html. Accessed January 11, 2018.

33. MacArthur Foundation. Jeffrey Brenner. Available at: https://www.macfound.org/fellows/886/. Accessed January 11, 2018.

34. Camden Coalition of Healthcare Providers. National Center for Complex Health and Social Needs website. Available at: https://www.camdenhealth.org/national-center/. Accessed January 11, 2018.

35. Beck AF, Sandel MT, Ryan PH, Kahn RS. Mapping neighborhood health geomarkers to clinical care decisions to promote equity in child health. *Health Affairs*. June 2017;36(6):1000.

36. Beck AF, Sandel MT, Ryan PH, Kahn RS. Mapping neighborhood health geomarkers to clinical care decisions to promote equity in child health. *Health Affairs*. June 2017;36(6):1000.

37. Young GJ, Chou C, Alexander JA, Lee SD, Raver E. Provision of community benefits by tax-exempt U.S. hospitals. *New England Journal of Medicine*. April 18, 2013;368(16):1519–1527; Crossley M, Tobin Tyler E, Herbst, J. Tax-exempt hospitals and community health under the Affordable Care Act: identifying and addressing unmet legal needs as social determinants of health. *Public Health Reports*. January-February 2016;131(1):195–199.

38. U.S. Department of the Treasury. Additional requirements for charitable hospitals; community health needs assessments for charitable hospitals; requirement of a section 4959 excise tax return and time for filing the return. *Federal Register*. 2014;79:78954.

39. Luthra S. Nonprofit hospitals focused more on community needs under the ACA. That may change. *The Washington Post*. March 14, 2017. https://www.washingtonpost.com/national /health-science/nonprofit-hospitals-focused-more-on-community-needs-under-the-aca -that-may-change/2017/03/14/4214f3fe-080c-11e7-b77c-0047d15a24e0_story.html?utm _term=.a12bab6f29c3.

40. Blue Cross Blue Shield of Massachusetts Foundation. Leveraging the social determinants of health: what works? June 2015. Available at: https://bluecrossmafoundation.org/sites/default /files/download/publication/Social_Equity_Report_Final.pdf.

41. Abrams M, Moulds D. Integrating medical and social services: a pressing priority for health systems and payers. *Health Affairs Blog*. July 5, 2015. Available at: http://www.healthaffairs .org/do/10.1377/hblog20160705.055717/full/. Accessed January 11, 2018.

42. Centers for Medicare and Medicaid Services. Accountable health communities. Available at: https://innovation.cms.gov/initiatives/ahcm. Accessed January 11, 2018.

43. Crawford M, Houston R. State payment and financing models to promote health and social service integration. Center for Health Care Strategies (brief); 2015. Available at: https:// www.chcs.org/resource/state-payment-financing-models-promote-health-social-service -integration/. Accessed January 11, 2018.

44. Bachrach D, Guyer J, Levin A. Medicaid coverage of social interventions: a road map for states. Milbank Memorial Fund (issue brief); July 2016: 12. Available at: https://www.milbank.org /publications/medicaid-coverage-social-interventions-road-map-states/. Accessed January 11, 2018.

45. Katz MH. Homelessness—challenges and progress. *The JAMA Network*. Viewpoint. Published online, October 31, 2017. Available at: https://jamanetwork.com/journals/jama /fullarticle/2661031. Accessed January 11, 2018.

46. Sandel M, Desmond M. Investing in housing for health improves both mission and margin. *The JAMA Network*. Viewpoint. Published online October 31, 2017. Available at: https:// jamanetwork.com/journals/jama/fullarticle/2661030. Accessed January 11, 2018.

47. Institute of Medicine. For the public's health: revitalizing law and policy to meet new challenges; 2011: 12. Available at: http://www.nationalacademies.org/hmd/Reports/2012/For -the-Publics-Health-Investing-in-a-Healthier-Future.aspx. Accessed January 11, 2018.

48. Public Health Institute and the American Public Health Association. Health in All Policies: a guide for state and local governments; 2013: 6. Available at: http://www.phi.org /resources/?resource=hiapguide. Accessed January 11, 2018.

49. The National Prevention and Health Promotion Strategy. The National Prevention Strategy: America's plan for better health and wellness; June 2011. Available at: https://www .surgeongeneral.gov/priorities/prevention/strategy/index.html. Accessed January 11, 2018.

50. Public Health Institute and the American Public Health Association. Health in All Policies: a guide for state and local governments; 2013: 7. Available at: http://www.phi.org /resources/?resource=hiapguide. Accessed January 11, 2018.

51. The Centers for Disease Control and Prevention. Health impact assessments. Available at: https://www.cdc.gov/healthyplaces/hia.htm. Accessed January 11, 2018.

52. Mattessich PW, Rausch EJ. Cross-sector collaboration to improve community health: a view of the current landscape. *Health Affairs.* 2014;33(11):1968–1974.

53. Change Lab Solutions. Healthier communities through redevelopment: rebuilding neighborhoods for better nutrition and active living; 2012. Available at: http://www .changelabsolutions.org/publications/healthier-redevelopment. Accessed January 11, 2018.

54. Prevention Institute. Tool for Health & Resilience In Vulnerable Environments (THRIVE). Available at: https://www.preventioninstitute.org/tools/thrive-tool-health-resilience -vulnerable-environments. Accessed January 11, 2018.

55. National Center for Medical-Legal Partnership. The need. Available at: http://medical -legalpartnership.org/need/. Accessed January 11, 2018.

56. National Center for Medical-Legal Partnership. Partnerships. Available at: http://medical -legalpartnership.org/partnerships/. Accessed January 11, 2018.

57. National Center for Medical-Legal Partnership. Impact. Available at: http://medical -legalpartnership.org/impact/.

58. Plumb JD, Plumb E, Roy V, Salzman B. Population health education. In: Nash DB, Fabius RJ, Skoufalos A, et al., eds. *Population Health: Creating a Culture of Wellness.* Burlington, MA: Jones & Bartlett Learning; 2015: 61.

59. Gonzalo JD, Skochelak SE, Wolpaw DR. Health systems science in medical education. In: Skochelak SE, Hawkins RE, Lawson LE, et al., eds. *Health Systems Science.* Philadelphia, PA: Elsevier; 2017: 5.

60. Gonzalo JD, Skochelak SE, Wolpaw DR. Health systems science in medical education. In: Skochelak SE, Hawkins RE, Lawson LE, et al., eds. *Health Systems Science.* Philadelphia, PA: Elsevier; 2017: 5.

61. Tobin Tyler E, Rodgers M, Weintraub, D. Bridging the health and legal professions through education and training. In: Tobin Tyler E, Lawton E, Conroy C, et al., eds. *Poverty, Health and Law: Readings and Cases for Medical-Legal Partnership.* Durham, NC: Carolina Academic Press; 2012: 97–123.

62. Mullan F. Social mission in health professions education: beyond Flexner. *JAMA.* July 11, 2017;318(2):123.

63. Sharma M, Pinto AD, Kumagai AK. Teaching the social determinants of health: a path to equity or a road to nowhere? *Academic Medicine.* January 2018; 93(10):25-30.

64. Metzl J, Hansen H. Structural competency: theorizing a new medical engagement with stigma and inequality. *Social Science & Medicine.* 2014;103:128–131.

65. Sukhera J, Watling C. A framework for integrating implicit bias recognition into health professions education. *Academic Medicine.* January 2018;93(10):35–40.

66. Sukhera J, Watling C. A framework for integrating implicit bias recognition into health professions education. *Academic Medicine.* January 2018;93(10):35–40.

67. Sukhera J, Watling C. A framework for integrating implicit bias recognition into health professions education. *Academic Medicine.* January 2018;93(10):35–40.

CHAPTER 7

Advocating for Health Justice: What You Can Do

▶ Introduction

In other chapters, we have presented many factors, both within and outside the health care system, that contribute to health inequity—insufficient government support for people's basic human needs, including health care services; historical and extant discrimination affecting marginalized groups; and other social and structural barriers to health and the inadequacy of current laws and policies in addressing those barriers. With the seeming intransigence of health and health care disparities, you may be asking yourself, "What can I do to make a difference?" In the chapter on creating holistic systems to care for socially complex patients and populations, we described some of the recent efforts, driven by health system reform and the relatively new focus on the social determinants of health (SDOH), to better integrate and improve access to health services for patients and families and promote intersectoral approaches to health equity. In this chapter, we explore how health care, public health, social service, and legal professionals can advocate for changes that promote health justice.

As we describe, advocacy can span from helping and empowering individual patients to access the health care, social, and legal services they need, to insisting on health and other stakeholder system changes in order to reduce barriers to health for vulnerable populations, to partnering with community members to effect policy change at the local, state, and federal levels. Recognizing some of the political, professional, and systems barriers to achieving health justice, we explore some of the skills and strategies necessary for success.

▶ Defining Advocacy

The term *advocacy* has broad meaning across many different contexts, so it is worth defining it before beginning our exploration of how it applies to health justice. Let's start with this definition: "[A]s an action or practice, advocacy as a generic term is used in a much more general sense to describe actions that support or empower individuals or groups. On a broad continuum, advocacy can range from representing others to self-advocacy, where individuals either take their own actions or are supported to speak for themselves through information or education."[1] We like this definition because it acknowledges that advocacy is not always about one person speaking on behalf of another or a group, but also includes supporting people to speak for themselves. As we discuss the roles of professionals in advocacy, keep in mind that advocates should always be cognizant of the power dynamics and pitfalls involved in speaking for others.

▶ Health Advocacy — *Physician advocacy* *Public health advocacy*

Much has been written about the role of health professionals as advocates. Consider this definition of *physician advocacy* from Earnest and colleagues: "Action by a physician to promote those social, economic, educational, and political changes that ameliorate the suffering and threats to human health and well-being that he or she identifies through his or her professional work and expertise."[2] On the other hand, *public health advocacy* has been defined as: "[A]dvocacy that is intended to reduce death or disability in groups of people (overall or from a specific cause) and that is not confined to clinical settings. Such advocacy involves the use of information and resources to reduce the occurrence or severity of public health problems."[3] Both of these definitions pertaining to health advocacy focus on ways in which health care and public health professionals can help to identify and argue for community-level changes (inside and outside the clinical context) that are likely to improve the health of patients and populations. Obviously, health advocacy is not limited to health care and public health professionals. Social workers, nurses, community health workers, lawyers, and other professionals, as well as patients and community members, advocate on behalf of individuals and for systems and policy changes intended to improve health.

We explore below four critical questions that arise in health advocacy: (1) What is the professional responsibility of health care providers and other health professionals to engage in advocacy beyond addressing the individual needs of patients or clients? (2) What are the goals of advocacy efforts in the context of health justice? (3) What types of advocacy efforts are likely to be effective in promoting health equity and justice? and (4) What skills and strategies lend themselves to effective health justice advocacy? As we explore these questions, keep this final point about health advocacy in mind: "Advocacy should ultimately be aiming to remedy injustices, not simply to make those injustices more bearable. This means that advocacy will be generally aiming to bring about the sort of social and structural change that will give people… a more integral and pivotal place in all the many environments in which people live, work and interact."[4]

▶ Professional Roles and Responsibilities

With the growing focus in health care on SDOH, health professions educators have increasingly argued that professional training should include advocacy skills. But why should health professionals be expected to embrace advocacy as part of their professional roles? Some point to professional ethical guidelines as providing justification for this expectation. For example, the American Medical Association's (AMA) *Declaration of Professional Responsibility: Medicine's Social Contract With Humanity* states that physicians pledge to "advocate for social, economic, educational and political changes that ameliorate suffering and contribute to human well-being."[5] The definition of advocacy offered by Earnest and colleagues above clearly builds on the AMA declaration. There is disagreement, however, about the extent of a physician's obligation to engage in advocacy. Some argue that advocacy is a noble endeavor, but should be considered an optional activity for physicians with a particular interest in it.[6] In contrast, others view medicine as a social contract in which "society grants the medical professions—comprising individuals and their collective associations—special social status and certain privileges such as monopoly use of knowledge, practice autonomy, and the right to self-regulate. In return, the medical profession is expected to promote society's health."[7]

Beyond the debate about whether advocacy should be required of physicians is the question of whether physicians are likely to be effective advocates, particularly when compared to other professionals, such as lawyers and public health professionals, who may be better trained and thus more skilled. One answer to this question is that people listen to physicians and other health professionals more than they do to others. In a recent Gallup poll, nurses, pharmacists, and doctors were the top three rated professions for honesty and ethical standards.[8] As we discuss below, health professionals are in a particularly strong position to articulate the needs of vulnerable patients and populations and to advocate for systems and policy changes that support health justice.

Ethical guidelines for public health practice promote advocacy as a core responsibility as well: "Public health should advocate and work for the empowerment of disenfranchised community members, aiming to ensure that the basic resources and conditions necessary for health are accessible to all."[9] Ethical codes for social workers, nurses, and lawyers all speak to their obligation to, in some way, advocate for underserved populations and promote social justice. But what are the best ways for professionals who are committed to health equity and justice to advocate for changes that will improve the lives of individuals, families, and communities?

Just as there is great benefit in developing interprofessional and intersectoral partnerships for more effective and better coordinated service delivery to vulnerable populations, partnerships across sectors are critically important for effective advocacy. Medical-legal partnerships (MLP) (described in the chapter on creating holistic systems to care for socially complex patients and populations) have shown the value of bringing together health professionals and lawyers to advocate for systems and policy changes:

> Health care providers who engage in MLP are more likely to understand the interaction between social and legal systems and patient health. By working closely with an attorney, physicians, nurses and other members of the health care team can gain insight into the laws, policies, and regulations that affect patient health and well-being. They can discover legal remedies that can be taken to amend and improve an ineffective policy.[10]

Because lawyers are trained to challenge systems and to identify the ways in which laws and policies may adversely affect people, they bring a skill set that is extremely helpful to health advocacy efforts. Similarly, collaboration between public health professionals and lawyers can support thoughtful public health laws and policies that "drive the provision of public health services toward those in greatest need."[11] By bringing together professionals with unique perspectives and expertise, interprofessional advocacy efforts are more likely to bring about sustainable systems change.

▶ Goals and Strategies of Health Justice Advocacy

Thus far, we have described the *why* and the *who* of health advocacy: why it's important for professionals with specific ethical obligations, expertise, and skill sets to engage in advocacy to improve systems, laws, and policies that benefit patient and population health. Now we turn to the *what* and the *how*: what are the types of goals and strategies involved in health advocacy and how can health professionals and their partners most effectively engage in health advocacy when there may be significant barriers to doing so?

Because there are different levels of advocacy with (potentially) their own disparate goals and strategies, we start this section by delineating three levels of advocacy: individual advocacy (i.e., advocacy on behalf of an individual patient or family); health systems advocacy (which focuses on changing institutional practice); and local, state, and federal policy advocacy. Note that an important distinction is the difference between advocating on behalf of a patient by helping him or her to navigate systems to better access needed resources and services, and advocating for changes to those systems to better serve a larger patient population. One author describes this distinction as the difference between health care providers as *agents* versus health care providers as *activists*. In the former, providers *work the system*; in the latter they work to *change the system*.[12] While both of these roles are important, they have different goals.

Individual Advocacy

Health care, social service, and legal professionals are all trained to identify needs of individual patients or clients and to help them navigate systems in order to achieve their goals. In the case of health care providers, when they act as the patient's agent, they "act on a patient's behalf in order to secure access to resources, facilities, and support (such as specialist care, diagnostic testing, and ancillary services). This role, therefore, involves supporting the individual patient in his or her journey through health."[13] As we discussed in the chapter on creating holistic systems to care for socially complex patients and populations, some health care providers are now being trained and expected to identify and address their patients' social needs as part of improving the quality of health care delivery. Many would argue that this type of individual advocacy by health care providers is a fundamental part of their professional obligation and fiduciary duty to their patients. But helping patients access the resources and services they need also requires that providers recognize and support patients' own agency in their health. To advocate for patients without adequately engaging them in decision making and empowering them to navigate systems on their own behalf creates the danger of paternalism. Patient engagement in their own health and the systems with which they interact is a critical component of advocacy. Patient and family engagement can be defined as "patients, families, their representatives, and health professionals working in active partnership at various levels across the health care system—direct care, organizational design and governance, and policy making—to improve health and health care."[14]

While individual advocacy is part and parcel of quality health care, providers can become frustrated and burned out if they fight the same battles over and over again, patient after patient. These battles may have to do with systemic problems in health care delivery (such as poor access to language services for non-English speaking patients) or with policy failures (e.g., inadequate supports for families with food insecurity). Health care providers and administrators are often in the best position to identify system and policy failures that lead to poor health outcomes and health disparities. Advocacy at the institutional and policy levels is the most effective way to make changes that will result in better population health. Focusing on how systems and policies fail vulnerable populations is particularly critical, as they are the populations most likely to be negatively affected by inadequate or poorly enforced policies and the ones with the least power to effectuate change.

Institutional Advocacy

When thinking about systems change, one's focus often goes to changing laws and policies (and we discuss the importance of legal and policy change below). But institutional practices and protocols can also create enormous barriers to effective delivery of care and to helping patients access vital resources and services that impact their health. In the chapter on creating holistic systems to care for socially complex patients and populations, we described the many ways in which health institutions can implement systems changes targeted at improving the health of vulnerable populations—e.g., screening for health-related social needs, building community partnerships with social services, and targeting resources to the most vulnerable patient populations. How can health care providers, administrators, and their partners initiate change within their own institutions to better serve vulnerable populations? In some ways, institutional advocacy may be the most difficult type in that it often requires individuals to confront their superiors and to challenge the status quo. The recent focus on health care quality improvement has highlighted the challenges of organizational change.[15]

In the context of improving health care and social service delivery to vulnerable populations, advocates often find that they are met with the competing priorities of health care institutions. Health care institutions often cite lack of resources and budget cuts as reasons for failing to implement systems changes designed to better serve vulnerable patients. For example, hiring a social worker or community health worker or creating a medical-legal partnership may be viewed as a luxury when a hospital is losing money. Despite legal requirements under Title VI of the 1964 Civil Rights Act that federally subsidized health care facilities provide appropriate interpretation services for non-English speaking patients, many facilities have woefully inadequate services. How can health professionals and their partners effectively advocate for institutional change, particularly when it may mean confronting the bureaucracies in which they work?

For effective institutional advocacy, we offer three suggestions. First, there is power in numbers. An individual health care provider may have difficulty persuading leadership that a social worker, MLP, or interpreter service is crucial to quality care for patients. However, a group of providers with the same message is likely to be a much more powerful voice. Multiple providers who can articulate in a unified voice the impact on patient care of failing to offer these services are much more likely to be successful than an advocate who goes it alone. Second, persistent advocacy may pay off over time. Persuading leadership that change is needed or new resources are required may be initially met with rejection, but persistent advocacy can help to, over time, move the issue to the top of the priority list. Third, start small and build from small successes. The best way to make the case for change is to demonstrate the importance of that change. For example, you may not be able to convince a hospital administrator to fund a full-time community health worker but she or he may be willing to pilot a half-time position. Collecting data to show the importance and impact of this resource will make it easier to make the argument for additional resources in the future and to expand and sustain the resource over time.

Policy Advocacy

Before jumping into policy advocacy, it is helpful to first define and briefly discuss what we mean by "policy." Most of us associate policy with legislation, but there are multiple levers for creating and changing policy, in both private and public sector contexts. In the context of public policy, a good starting point is the following: "Generally, public policy can be defined as a system of laws, regulatory measures, courses of action and funding priorities concerning a given topic promulgated by a government entity or its representative."[16] The key here is that public policy can be thought of as a decision (or a series of decisions) made by government officials from the three branches of government—executive, legislative, and judicial—and at all levels—local, state, and federal. In a representative government like that in the United States, there are numerous ways in which citizens have an opportunity influence public policy. Here we offer a very brief overview of the process and terminology related to law and policymaking. We encourage you to learn more about this process from more detailed sources.

A *bill* is proposed legislation that articulates a change in policy, creates or modifies a program, or appropriates funding. The opportunities for advocacy throughout this process are numerous—from partnering with a legislator or his or her aide to draft the bill, to suggesting amendments, to arguing for its passage. Once a bill becomes law, it is referred to as a *statute*. Statutes are the laws passed by legislatures and signed into law by the executive leader at the federal, state, county, or city levels. Generally, statutes set out broad policy objectives but often lack detail about implementation and enforcement. These details are typically spelled out in *administrative regulations* that describe how the law will be carried out to promote the statute's policy goals. A federal or state administrative agency is charged with the task of writing these regulations. The process of creating federal or state regulations is generally referred to as the "rulemaking" process as depicted in **FIGURE 7.1**.

Like the legislative process, there are opportunities throughout the rulemaking process for advocates to weigh in—from providing the agency with evidence and information in the early stages when proposed regulations are being drafted, to alerting interested parties about the proposed regulations, to offering expert testimony during the comment period. Agencies are required to offer a comment period for any proposed regulation, so this is an excellent opportunity to influence the final rule. For example, advocacy by health care and public health professionals was instrumental in securing inclusion of certain population health provisions in the Affordable Care Act and the thousands of pages of regulations promulgated to implement that law.

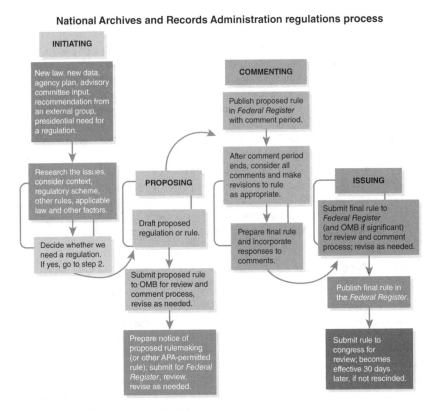

National Archives and Records Administration regulations process

FIGURE 7.1 The administrative rulemaking process.

From National Archives and Records Administration.

Thus, there are a variety of ways in which health and legal professionals and their partners concerned with health justice can engage in the legislative and rulemaking process to effect change:

- Formulating policy positions on specific bills
- Preparing and presenting testimony before legislative committees
- Providing public comment on agency rules and regulations
- Initiating telephone calls and writing e-mails or letters to concerned stakeholders to urge a particular action on specific or categorical legislation
- Sponsoring or holding meetings, furnishing speakers, or preparing and distributing pamphlets and other literature to stimulate reaction to legislation
- Circulating petitions, contacting legislators or participating in other efforts to impact legislative issues

In addition to helping to ensure that laws and regulations are created with health justice in mind, it is also important to not lose focus on how existing laws are implemented and enforced once all the legal text has been written. In the chapter on existing safety net programs and legal protections, we discussed some of the health consequences of the lack of enforcement of existing laws, such as poor enforcement of housing safety codes and protective orders for victims of intimate partner violence. Government actors charged with enforcing the law must be held accountable in order to ensure that people are protected in the ways envisioned in the written law. Yet, bureaucracies often fail to hold up this end of the bargain and people experiencing challenging life circumstances are usually not in a good position to fight for their rights on their own. Health professionals working in partnership with community organizers and lawyers can be extremely effective in exposing enforcement failures and advocating for more accountability by government actors. An example of this type of partnership is the Breathe Easy at Home program, initiated by Boston Medical Center. Pediatric providers, frustrated by substandard housing conditions leading to asthma exacerbations in their patients, met with officials from the Housing Inspection Division in Boston, Massachusetts and with public health officials to strategize about how to implement more timely enforcement. They designed a shared website allowing health providers to directly refer patients with asthma for housing inspections when they suspect that housing conditions are triggering a child's asthma. Direct communication between the Housing Inspection Division and health care providers has led to more timely response to health harming housing conditions.[17]

Local Policy Advocacy

While policy at the state or federal level is more likely to effect change for a greater number of people, there is much to be said for engaging in policy advocacy at the local level. First, policy change at the local level is often easier to achieve in a short amount of time. Advocates are more likely to have access to decision makers and to be able to make their voices heard by testifying at city council or mayoral meetings. They are also in a better position to hold government officials accountable for policy failures or poor enforcement by directly transmitting information about the barriers their patients or clients experience. Second, as we discussed earlier, advocacy is most effective when it engages multiple constituencies by creating effective coalitions. Although there are certainly effective state and federal level coalitions working toward health and social policy change, community coalitions can best empower members of the community affected by policy to shape sustainable change. In promoting health justice, it is particularly important that health advocates not usurp power from vulnerable populations. Instead, they can provide information in support of the agenda driven by the community and help to facilitate multisector coalition building.

Finally, with regard to changing policy to address the SDOH, local policy can be very effective in changing the environments in which people live. The Praxis Project, a nonprofit organization focused on building "healthy communities by transforming the power relationships and structures that affect our lives,"[18] notes that:

> Local policy work deserves more attention, not only for its local impact but because *it is now the primary form in which social policy is developed*. Policy development, previously the domain of experts and lobbyists, is increasingly being used as a tool for community change. Grassroots groups are taking their own agendas to city hall and the state house and proactively transforming them into progressive, meaningful policies.[19]

A whole range of local policies can improve population health and promote health equity, such as laws and policies raising the minimum wage, zoning liquor and grocery stores, and structuring public transportation routes. In addition, local policy changes are often precursors to state policy changes. By providing evidence of a health benefit to the community, local policies can help bolster arguments for change at the state and federal policy levels.

State Policy Advocacy

Advocating at the state policy level, like the local level, has a number of advantages. Because state legislators' constituencies are smaller than those of members of the U.S. Congress, state policymakers are much more accessible and often more willing to meet individually with advocates to hear their concerns. Unlike in Congress, where advocates must be invited to offer testimony in support or opposition to a bill, in state legislatures, citizens can generally sign up to testify on a bill of interest. Health care providers and public health advocates are in a unique position to offer information about the disparate impact of particular policies on vulnerable populations using data and patient anecdotes.

Additionally, because health care and safety net programs are usually administered at the state level, administrative advocacy is critical to changes in policy and practices that can significantly benefit vulnerable populations. For example, in Rhode Island, advocates helped to secure Medicaid funding for nonmedical services for lead-poisoned children and their families.[20] (The chapter on creating holistic systems to care for socially complex patients and populations provides other examples of state Medicaid program innovations focused on addressing SDOH.) Advocates can also challenge ineffective state administration of safety net programs—such as the SNAP, WIC, TANF, and Section 8 housing subsidy programs—that can lead to unnecessary food and housing insecurity. Again, health care providers in partnership with public health, legal and social service partners can be very effective advocates for policy change and enforcement by demonstrating the health impact of these failures on vulnerable populations.

Federal Policy Advocacy

With the ongoing dysfunction and gridlock in Congress, it may be tempting to write off the benefit of federal policy advocacy. But obviously, ceding advocacy efforts to the powerful interests that tend to control the policy levers in Washington, DC would do a huge disservice to disenfranchised populations. The successful efforts in 2017 to beat back attempts to repeal the Affordable Care Act and to significantly reduce Medicaid funding speaks to the importance and power of advocacy (which, as seen in both of these examples, is often needed just to maintain existing legal protections and programs). Because attempting to influence federal policy can appear overwhelming, we outline briefly some of the ways in which advocates can make a difference.

As described earlier, there are many entry points for influencing proposed legislation and regulations. While it may be more difficult to testify on a particular bill being heard by a congressional committee rather than by a state legislative body, you should not discount the opportunity to lobby your member of Congress or to submit comments on proposed federal regulations on an issue about which you are concerned. Members of Congress spend time in their home districts and most have legislative aides who focus on various matters pertaining to health policy. Identifying the appropriate contact in the legislator's district office and scheduling a time to discuss an issue or a particular bill can be very valuable in drawing the legislator's attention to the issue or bill and potentially swaying his or her vote. Most members of Congress value input from health advocates, particularly when the advocate can offer new information, data, or a different perspective on the topic or bill. Similarly, as described above, administrative agencies seek out comments from individuals and organizations that bring expertise to a particular issue during the rulemaking process. For example, women's health advocates have played a critical role in lobbying Congress to repeal the Trump Administration rules allowing employers to deny health insurance coverage for birth control methods based on religious objections. (The new administrative rules reverse the contraceptive mandate set forth in the Affordable Care Act).

But federal advocacy is not only about weighing in on the drafting of bills or rules, it is frequently about budget appropriations. The federal budget represents the values of the government and unfortunately, those values usually do not prioritize funding for efforts to promote health justice. In 2017, President Trump's budget, titled "A New Foundation for American Greatness," proposed deep cuts in programs affecting vulnerable populations, including $800 billion from Medicaid, $192 billion from food assistance, $272 billion from welfare programs, and $72 billion from disability benefits.[21] Since Congress—rather than the president—has the authority to pass the final budget for the nation, advocates can play a large role in lobbying against these types of cuts and providing evidence regarding their consequences for the health and well-being of vulnerable populations.

To feel less overwhelmed and isolated in advocating for federal policy change, individual advocates should work with partners by either helping to build coalitions in their own communities around a particular issue or by supporting the work of established advocacy organizations. Advocacy organizations that focus on improving health care access for the underserved, reducing health disparities, and/or promoting social justice seek members and partners that share their goals and who can support their agendas with different types of evidence, information, and perspectives. In particular, many welcome support and participation by health professionals who speak to the health impact of issues that may not traditionally be viewed as health policy issues. For example, gun control advocates have increasingly sought the support of health care providers and public health experts who can speak to the individual toll, as well as the epidemiological data, stemming from gun violence.

Before turning to some of the specific skills and strategies involved in effective advocacy, it is worth reiterating that policy advocacy that is done in a vacuum—i.e., without engaging the community affected—is not only less effective in making lasting change, it is also less likely to fundamentally challenge the power structures that drive disempowerment of vulnerable populations. Health and legal professionals have much to offer (knowledge, expertise, experience, and passion) in advocating for health justice. But it is important to keep in mind that advocacy must be driven by listening to the daily concerns and experiences of patients and constituents and working to not only change systems and policies affecting their health, but also to challenge the systems that keep their voices from being heard.

▶ Skills for Effective Health Justice Advocacy

Developing advocacy skills takes time and experience. For professionals new to advocacy, identifying and cultivating relationships with mentors who are effective advocates in your community can be helpful in avoiding common mistakes. Additionally, listening to patients, clients, and community members about the injustices they experience and tracking patterns in your practice that point to system and policy failures are critical steps to take before jumping into an advocacy strategy. Below we offer some of the skills and relevant questions associated with developing an advocacy strategy.

1. Recognizing opportunities for advocacy
   - Have you listened to the concerns of patients and others in your community?
   - What issues are other health advocates focusing on and why?
   - What systems or policy barriers and failures can you identify that create inequity in health care access or health outcomes for the patients or clients you serve?
2. Building sustainable relationships with community partners, advocacy organizations, legislators, and media
   - Who can you work with to develop your strategy and achieve your goals?
   - Who is already working on the issue in your community and how can you support those efforts?
3. Defining your goal and your audience
   - What are you trying to achieve (passage of legislation, regulatory change, budget appropriation, change within your health care institution) and why?
   - What decision maker should you target to make this change and how can you persuade him or her that the change is needed?
4. Developing and sticking to your message
   - Is your message clearly defined with a specific "ask"?
   - Are you and your advocacy partners consistent in your messaging?
5. Crafting compelling stories to frame your issue
   - Are there anecdotes and/or data that can help decision makers to understand why the system or policy change is needed?
   - Can you articulate the effect of the system or policy issue on real people?

The most critical first step in an advocacy strategy is to identify allies and to build consensus among partners about what you are trying to achieve and why. Grassroots advocacy requires that diverse voices are heard, but to be effective, those voices must be aligned around a common and consistent message. Advocacy is a team sport. Before undertaking an advocacy effort, it is important to build relationships with people from the community as well as allies who can help deliver the message in a compelling way, including people from the media and supportive legislators. Two common mistakes that advocates make are to not spend sufficient time building relationships and failing to get on the same page with other advocates. This can lead to embarrassment and failure if legislators perceive that advocates do not have a clear message or shared goals.

Another common pitfall in advocacy is to set goals too high. Passionate advocates want to see change and they want it to happen fast. But systems and policy change generally move extremely slow. Pacing yourself while maintaining your persistence will help you to stay engaged and not give up if you do not achieve your goals quickly. It can take several years for proposed legislation to even be heard in committee, let alone pass and become law. The history of health care reform is a helpful reminder of the pace of policy change—Theodore Roosevelt first proposed a social insurance plan in 1912, which would have included health insurance.[22] It might also be said that advocacy is an endurance sport. Setting short-term, attainable goals and benchmarks can help advocates play the long game and not become discouraged.[23] Doctor Thomas O'Toole, a physician-advocate, highlights the personal "do's" and "don'ts" for clinician-advocates working toward health justice in **TABLE 7.1**.

TABLE 7.1 Do's and Don'ts of Clinician Advocacy

Do's	Don'ts
Know your issue.	Don't become bigger than your issue. A little humility can go a long way.
Know who is involved.	Don't isolate or let your cause consume you.
Develop your skills.	Don't assume that your medical training is adequate.
Partner, organize, and build coalitions.	Don't be a "lone ranger" in your advocacy.
Be strategic; set benchmarks and realistic goals.	Don't forget what you want to do, and why you are doing it.

Data from O'Toole TP. Advocacy. In: King TE, Wheeler MB, et al., *Medical Management of Vulnerable and Underserved Populations*. New York: McGraw Hill; 2007: 433.

TABLE 7.2 Episodic vs. Longitudinal Advocacy Activities

Episodic	Longitudinal
■ Write a letter to the editor. ■ Publish an opinion piece for traditional media, social media, or health professional journal. ■ Call or write to a legislator. ■ Testify at a hearing. ■ Meet with an elected official. ■ Prepare a news brief. ■ Donate money to a campaign or individual. ■ Vote. ■ Participate in or organize a voter registration drive. ■ Phone bank on an issue. ■ Start or join a social media campaign, create a website. ■ Host a fundraiser for a candidate for office.	■ Run for elected office. ■ Conduct research on policy-related science. ■ Serve as a health advisor to a legislator or media contact. ■ Teach advocacy skills to students in the health professions. ■ Serve on the board of directors for a professional or community organization. ■ Form a community coalition. ■ Take a leadership role in your professional society. ■ Lead a health care organization.

Data from Choi RY, Gottlieb L, Chen AH. Advocacy. In: King TE, et al., *Medical Management of Vulnerable and Underserved Patients: Principles, Practice and Populations*. New York: McGraw Hill; 2016: 83.

It is also important to remember that advocacy activities are extremely varied, ranging from writing letters to a newspaper editor to leading an advocacy organization. **TABLE 7.2** demonstrates how these activities can be episodic or longitudinal. The important thing is to identify ways to engage in advocacy around issues that you are passionate about and that are driven by your understanding of and experiences with health injustice.

▶ Framing the Need for Change

One of the greatest challenges of health justice advocacy is framing the need for systems and policy change within a political context that is often deaf to the dignity and needs of vulnerable populations. As we discussed earlier in the text, the U.S. has a uniquely individualistic and market-driven approach to social policy, including health policy. Because health care is generally viewed as a market commodity, rather than a service that the government is obliged to provide its citizens, persuading policymakers that the government has a responsibility for improving the conditions in which vulnerable people live can be difficult. Similarly, as we described earlier, notions about the deserving and undeserving poor continue to influence support for safety net programs, and Americans are deeply divided by political party with regard to government responsibility for helping the disadvantaged. See **FIGURE 7.2**.

Recognizing the extreme political polarization in the U.S., public health lawyer and professor Gene Matthews and his colleagues argue that public health advocates need to reconsider the ways in which they have typically framed their policy arguments:

> Public health has tended to frame its policy arguments and legal foundations through the lens of liberal values for the last few decades. Opportunities are missed because public health hesitates in recognizing how to frame our messaging in a richer way that appeals to a broader spectrum of moral concerns. We argue that, particularly in these turbulent times, public health needs to examine more carefully how to frame its messages.[24]

Citing Jon Haidt's book, *The Righteous Mind: Why Good People Are Divided by Politics and Religion*, they argue that health advocates need to reframe arguments to take into consideration the moral values that shape both liberal and conservative perspectives on policy, including the understanding that intuition based on these values shapes views more than reasoning does. Thus, "if our messages don't initially trigger favorable intuitive responses, they will be unheard no matter how rational and well-crafted."[25] Health advocates have focused their arguments on "liberal-favored" values like care, liberty, and fairness, usually ignoring values that resonate with conservatives, such as loyalty, authority, and sanctity.[26] In our polarized political world, advocates may need to develop new strategies and messages if they are going to be successful in promoting health justice through policy and systems change.

Another critical question for medical and public health professionals who engage in policy advocacy is: what evidence is most effective in persuading policymakers and the public that a particular policy change is warranted? Since many

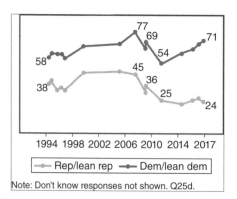

FIGURE 7.2 Views of increased government aid by political party.

health professionals are scientists, they often rely on scientific evidence and data to demonstrate the problem and need for change. But as we highlighted above, political will is often shaped by intuition, not necessarily rational arguments supported with data. This is not to argue that advocates should avoid using sound evidence to construct and support their policy arguments. It is, however, important to consider how data can be combined with stories and anecdotes that help the public and policymakers understand the human impact of a particular policy or policy failure. Patient stories can be extremely helpful in "tearing at the heartstrings" of the public and policymakers. For example, individual stories of cancer patients unable to acquire health insurance were used in the media by advocates to persuade policymakers that there was a need for expanded access to health insurance through the Affordable Care Act.

On the other hand, it is also important to recognize how individual stories and anecdotes can be used to paint a negative picture of particular groups of people, even when the evidence suggests that these anecdotes do not represent the majority of people in that group. During the 1980s, for example, President Ronald Reagan used the stereotype of the black "welfare queen" to persuade the public and other policymakers that the Aid to Families with Dependent Children (welfare) program was being abused by recipients (particularly black mothers) and that taxpayer dollars were being wasted. The "welfare queen" was depicted this way by Reagan:

> She has eighty names, thirty addresses, twelve Social Security cards and is collecting veteran's benefits on four non-existing deceased husbands. And she is collecting Social Security on her cards. She's got Medicaid, getting food stamps, and she is collecting welfare under each of her names. Her tax-free cash income is over $150,000.[27]

Despite the lack of evidence that mothers receiving welfare benefits were abusing the program this way, this anecdote was extremely powerful in moving the public and policymakers to believe that the welfare program was creating laziness and dependency among the poor, and that taxpayers were footing the bill. The title of the welfare reform law passed in 1996 indicates the power this welfare queen depiction had; it was titled "The Personal Responsibility and Work Opportunity Act." **TABLE 7.3** shows the pros and cons of anecdotes versus scientific evidence in advocating for policy change.

Framing persuasive arguments about the policy failures that lead to health inequity is complex. Ultimately, advocates rely on a range of narratives. While some advocates choose to focus on a value-based argument that health is a human right and the government has responsibility to support its citizens' basic needs, others rely on the more pragmatic economic argument that prevention (through health care and social services) will reduce downstream costs in health care spending (thereby saving taxpayers money). Both approaches, and others, may be needed for short- and long-term policy change. Advocates must decide what strategies they believe will be most effective in bringing about the change they seek.

TABLE 7.3 Understanding Anecdotes and Evidence in Public Policy

	Definition	Justification	Purpose
Anecdotes	Stories told to illustrate a problem or the failure of a policy, such as "I saw someone buy a steak with food stamps" or "welfare queen" stories	To justify starting or stopping programs by providing an easily understood story with obvious conclusions and underlying normative or moral principles	Good for staking out a position on an issue or motivating people to believe a certain way; less useful as part of serious analysis because they do not delve deeply into how programs work
Evidence from scientific study	Conclusions reached through scientific study of a problem or of the outcomes of a policy	To justify starting or stopping programs by providing the most scientifically sound information that policymakers can use to make decisions	Much stronger than anecdotes in understanding how and why things work the way they do; however, results of scientific studies are seldom straightforward and are always accompanied by unanswered questions. Many policymakers lack the technical expertise to fully understand the degree of uncertainty inherent in scientific analysis.

T. Birkland, An Introduction to the Policy Process: Theories, Concepts, and Models of Public Policy Making. New York: M.E. Sharpe, Inc., 2005. Reproduced by permission of Taylor and Francis Group, LLC, a division of Informa plc

▶ Conclusion

Persistent advocacy in support of health justice is critical to changing the laws, policies, and systems that can either positively support or negatively impact the health of vulnerable populations. Achieving health justice is a full agenda for advocates, but persistent focus on remedying policy failures and promoting innovative solutions can bring about incremental change:

> While large-scale reform leading to just institutions is not a near-term probability, striving for fairer treatment of mothers and their children,

greater gender equity, less social exclusion and racism, more inclusive and supportive communities, better environmental stewardship, more accountable government and corporations, fairer employment practices, and physical and social environments more conducive to human activity is possible. Doing so is our surest path—in fact, our only path—to improving population health.[28]

In the 1960s civil rights leaders coined the phrase "keep your eyes on the prize" in recognition that change is slow and that it will only come with persistence and clear focus. Working with others with a common purpose, setting realistic goals, and maintaining one's passion and focus will help advocates play the long game of achieving health justice.

References

1. Drage J. New Zealand's National Health and Disability Advocacy Service: a successful model of advocacy. *Health and Human Rights.* June 2012;14(1):1–11.
2. Earnest MA, Wong SL, Federico SG. Physician advocacy: what is it and how do we do it? *Academic Medicine.* January 2010;85(1):63–67.
3. Christoffel KK. Public health advocacy: process and product. *American Journal of Public Health.* May 2000;90(5):722–726.
4. Parsons I. *Oliver Twist Has Asked for More: The Politics and Practice of Getting Justice for People with Disabilities.* Victoria, Australia: Villamanta Publishing Service; 1994: 40.
5. American Medical Association. Declaration of professional responsibility: medicine's social contract with humanity; 2002.
6. Kanter SL. On physician advocacy. *Academic Medicine.* September 2011;86(9):1059–1060.
7. Gruen RL, Pearson SD, Brennan TA. Physician-citizens—public roles and professional obligations. *JAMA.* January 2004;291(1):94–98.
8. Norman J. Americans rate healthcare providers high on honesty, ethics. *Gallup News.* December 19, 2016. Available at: http://news.gallup.com/poll/200057/americans-rate-healthcare-providers-high-honesty-ethics.aspx.
9. Public Health Leadership Society. Principles of the ethical practice of public health; 2002. Available at: https://www.apha.org/~/media/files/pdf/membergroups/ethics_brochure.ashx.
10. Sandel M, Keller D, Lawton E, et al. Medical-legal partnership: strategies for policy. In: Tobin Tyler E, Lawton E, Conroy C, et al., eds. *Poverty, Health and Law: Readings and Cases for Medical-Legal Partnership.* Durham, NC: Carolina Academic Press; 2012: 594.
11. Matthews G, Burris S, Ledford SL, Gunderson G, Baker EL. Crafting richer public health messages for a turbulent political environment. *Journal of Public Health Management and Practice.* July/August 2017;23(4):420–423.
12. Dobson S, Voyer S, Hubinette M, Regehr G. From the clinic to the community: the activities and abilities of effective health advocates. *Academic Medicine.* February 2015;90(2):214–220.
13. Dobson S, Voyer S, Hubinette M, Regehr G. From the clinic to the community: the activities and abilities of effective health advocates. *Academic Medicine.* February 2015;90(2):214–220.
14. Carman KL, Dardess P, Maurer M, et al. Patient and family engagement: a framework for understanding the elements and developing interventions and policies. *Health Affairs.* February 2013;32(2):223–231.
15. Dixon-Woods M, McNicol S, Martin G. Ten challenges in improving quality in healthcare: lessons from the Health Foundation's programme evaluations and relevant literature. *BMJ Quality and Safety.* 2012;21:876–884.
16. Sandel M, Keller D, Lawton E, et al. Medical-legal partnership: strategies for policy change. In: Tobin Tyler E, Lawton E, Conroy C, et al., eds. *Poverty, Health and Law: Readings and Cases for Medical-Legal Partnership.* Durham, NC: Carolina Academic Press; 2012: 581.
17. City of Boston. Breathe easy at home. Available at: https://www.boston.gov/civic-engagement/breathe-easy-home.

18. Praxis Project website. Available at: https://www.thepraxisproject.org/.

19. Praxis Project. Advocating for better policies. Available at: http://www.unnaturalcauses.org /assets/uploads/file/UC_PolicyAdvocacy.pdf.

20. National Center for Healthy Housing and the Milken Institute School of Public Health, George Washington University. Case studies in healthcare financing of healthy homes services: Medicaid reimbursement for lead follow-up services in Rhode Island; October 2015. Available at: http://www.nchh.org/Portals/0/Contents/Lead_RI_final.pdf.

21. Davis JH. Trump's budget cuts deeply into Medicaid and anti-poverty efforts. *The New York Times.* May 22, 2017. Available at: https://www.nytimes.com/2017/05/22/us/politics/trump -budget-cuts.html?_r=0.

22. Teitelbaum JB, Wilensky SE. *Essentials of Health Policy and Law.* 3rd ed. Burlington, MA: Jones & Bartlett Learning; 2017.

23. O'Toole TP. Advocacy. In: King TE, Wheeler MB, Bindman AB, et al., eds. *Medical Management of Vulnerable & Underserved Patients: Principles, Practice, and Populations.* New York, NY: McGraw Hill; 2007: 434.

24. Matthews G, Burris S, Ledford SL, et al. Crafting richer public health messages for a turbulent political environment. *Journal of Public Health Management and Practice.* July/August 2017;23(4):420–421.

25. Matthews G, Burris S, Ledford SL, et al. Crafting richer public health messages for a turbulent political environment. *Journal of Public Health Management and Practice.* July/August 2017;23(4):421.

26. Matthews G, Burris S, Ledford SL, et al. Crafting richer public health messages for a turbulent political environment. *Journal of Public Health Management and Practice.* July/August 2017;23(4):421.

27. Black R, Sprague, A. The rise and reign of the welfare queen. September 22, 2016. *New America Weekly.* Available at: https://www.newamerica.org/weekly/edition-135 /rise-and-reign-welfare-queen/.

28. Davidson A. *Social Determinants of Health: A Comparative Approach.* Vancouver, Ontario: Oxford University Press; 2014: 265–266.

Conclusion

We recognize that this text, taken as a whole, may not have been a comforting read. In fact, it may have left you feeling downright distressed or dejected. If so, we hope these feelings trigger in you a desire to bring about change. Bryan Stevenson, an internationally acclaimed public interest lawyer and the Executive Director of the Equal Justice Initiative in Montgomery, Alabama, often talks about the need to do uncomfortable things as a precursor to change. Because people are biologically programmed to do what's comfortable, it's easy for us all to place ourselves in environments and situations that are, subjectively speaking, well known and comfortable. Inertia and the status quo can, unsurprisingly, result. According to Stevenson, it is thus incumbent upon people who seek change to fight against norms and their own proclivities—in other words, to do uncomfortable things. Perhaps reading some part of this text was uncomfortable to you, because it challenged certain beliefs (implicit biases?) or exposed you to unsavory societal practices or legal infirmities of which you were unaware. If so, how will you react?

In organizing your thoughts about how you can help create environments—whether a classroom, a conference room, a boardroom, a health clinic, a neighborhood, a state, or someplace else—that promote health justice, it is instructive to look back at some of the key themes that emerged throughout this text. Chapter 1 highlighted the fact that extant legal doctrines—including some that have nothing to do with health per se—operate in ways that make it more difficult for people to thrive and reach their full health potential. In this regard, an important first step for the nation would be to effectively shear away a slab of the "no duty to treat" principle by implementing a non–market-based health financing system that treats access to health care as a human right.

Chapters 2, 3, and 4 were of a specific kind: Chapter 2 singled out discrimination and bias as determinants of health that have deep-seated and enduring effects on marginalized populations, both within and outside the health care system; Chapter 3 reviewed the myriad types of health disparities that currently plague the United States; and Chapter 4 focused broadly on the range of social and structural forces that contribute to health and health care disparities. Important themes from these chapters include the particularly destructive and durable character of structural discrimination, the multifactorial and bidirectional nature of the pathways between social influences and health disparities, and the ruinous effect that poverty can have on individual and community health. Because structural pathologies can be especially insidious—surviving as they do across centuries and sectors, as individuals and institutions pass down and reinforce privilege, wealth, and power among a relative few—they require a concerted and vigorous response. One place to start would be a research program that (1) investigates the relationship between structural discrimination and population health and (2) assesses which policy interventions would create the greatest benefit for those populations that continue to be most affected by structural pathologies.[1]

Chapter 5 reviewed the extent to which existing safety net programs and related laws and policies address the social barriers to good health. There is little doubt that safety net programs are critically important in helping vulnerable individuals and families survive above the poverty level by providing access to necessities like health care, nutritious food, and adequate housing. At the same time, many safety net programs reach only a portion of the people who need them, and a debate rages on about who is "deserving" of tax-funded government assistance. If you are looking for a way to hone your advocacy chops in the context of health justice, fighting to keep the safety net from fraying is a good place to start.

In Chapter 6 we highlighted efforts being undertaken in the health care and public health systems to better coordinate and integrate health and social services and to promote health equity for socially complex populations. This included a discussion of innovative intersectoral collaborations, such as medical-legal partnerships and "Health in All Policies" initiatives focused on upstream systems reform. This chapter linked with Chapter 7, which highlighted the need for persistent, strategic, and interprofessional advocacy in support of those for whom health justice remains a goal on the horizon.

—

There is little doubt that the United States, compared even to other developed nations, has, collectively speaking, unique political, social, and cultural attributes. Some of these attributes include limited governmental power, a belief in self-governance, capitalism, unprecedented wealth, a strong sense of individualism, and racial and ethnic diversity. These characteristics have much to offer. At the same time, they do not always serve to create an environment in which health equity can flourish. Consider the following:

- Susan Fiske and Shelley Taylor, two preeminent social psychologists working in the subfield of social cognition, have spent their professional careers trying to better understand how people initially process and store information about other people, and how individuals then apply that information in social situations. As part of their work, Fiske and Taylor scanned the brains of high-achieving people in the U.S. to ascertain how these high achievers processed information about poor people. They found that the scanned brains processed images of poor people as if they were things, rather than human beings.[2]

- In a 2017 study, researchers analyzed population surveys from 32 high- and middle-income countries to determine how Americans' acceptance of health and health care disparities stacked up against the views of people in other similarly situated political and/or economic contexts. They found that the U.S. is an outlier in the very large share of people who don't find it unfair that many people lack access to needed health care. As the authors put it: "Relatively low levels of moral discomfort over income-based health care disparities despite broad awareness of unmet need indicate more public tolerance for health care inequalities in the United States than elsewhere."[3]

- Thirty-two percent of blacks surveyed in 2017 said they had personally experienced racial discrimination at a physician's office or a health clinic. Twenty-two percent indicated that they have gone so far as to avoid seeking medical care out of concern about discrimination.
- Thirty-one of the eighty-five richest people in the world are from the U.S. Their combined net worth is just over $1 trillion. That trillion dollars represents one-eighteenth of the U.S. economy, which itself represents one-quarter of the entire global economy.
- In the U.S., children are the age group most likely to live in poverty. Why? Although we could point to many specific structural causes, at bottom the answer lies in politics. Children can't vote, and too frequently low-income parents don't vote; as a result, child poverty does not live near the top of the nation's political agenda. (For instance, as we were writing this book, federal funding for the Children's Health Insurance Program (CHIP) dried up. CHIP provides health insurance coverage to nearly 9 million children in families that earn too much to qualify for Medicaid but who cannot afford private coverage. The program costs the federal government approximately $14 billion annually, or about 0.35% of the federal budget. While Congress debated corporate tax cuts in the fall of 2017, the deadline to renew CHIP funding passed.)

Large-scale health justice—i.e., the development and equal application of laws, policies, and behaviors that are evenhanded with regard to and display genuine respect for every person's health and well-being—simply cannot be achieved in this environment. While the nation has the power to correct its own health inequities and inequalities, major systemic change is required. Education has an important role to play. To be sure, health professions education should be expanded and deepened to better train clinicians of all types in the social complexities that dominate the lives of low-income patient populations. But again, as you have learned, health justice encompasses far more than just access to high-quality, nondiscriminatory health care, and many jobs pertinent to health justice reside outside the confines of the health professions. As a result, higher education generally should become more adept at training students in the multiple dimensions of inequality and poor health. Among other things, this requires educational programming across academic disciplines. Because of the many different pathways to health inequities, the various stakeholders who together can lead the nation down a new path should be educated together as early as possible, to understand one another's professional language, interventions, and goals. It has to be said that law schools—our own training ground—are particularly siloed in their approach to education. Though lawyers are unsurpassed in their understanding of complex administrative, constitutional, and poverty law, they historically have been trained as downstream fixes to existing legal crises. Training lawyers from the outset as "upstreamists" and as part of a broader team would help immensely.

Change for the better would also require the shifting of resources. We've discussed this at multiple points but it bears repeating: the nation's social needs are outstripping available resources, while trillions of dollars are spent annually on medical care to address some of the very problems created by the lack of social spending. A shift in resources from medical to social care would be especially compelling where it was channeled into early childhood programming and toward people who have been caught in the cycle of intergenerational poverty.

Finally, a movement toward health justice requires policy making that at all levels addresses the devastating health effects of the nation's structural illnesses—economic, social, and environmental.[4] As one author notes:

> Meaningful progress in addressing health inequities requires complementary policies to reduce inequities in education, employment, housing, transportation, and public safety. The decision makers with the greatest power to shape health outcomes are not health workers: Instead, they work on school boards or in municipal government, legislative bodies, housing authorities, transit agencies, or the business sector. They are employers, developers, investors, banks, philanthropists, voters, and journalists.[5]

But the policy making has to involve more than just the shifting of financial resources, and more than just an acknowledgment that health equity requires a quiver with many different types of arrows. It must embrace an empathic and tolerant approach to governing that seeks to reverse the accumulated social disadvantage of minorities of all types—racial, ethnic, gender, income, and geographic[6]—and affirms that respect for all people is an essential condition of a just, and healthy, society.

References

1. Bailey ZD, Krieger N, Agénor M, Graves J, Linos N, Bassett MT. Structural racism and health inequities in the U.S.A.: evidence and interventions. *Lancet.* 2017;389:1453–1463.
2. Fiske ST, Taylor SE. *Social Cognition: From Brains to Culture.* London, UK: Sage Publications Ltd.; 2017.
3. Hero JO, Zaslavsky AM, Blendon RJ. The United States leads other nations in differences by income in perceptions of health and health care. *Health Affairs.* June 2017;36(6):1032–1040.
4. Benfer EA. Health justice: a framework (and call to action) for the elimination of health inequity and social justice. *American University Law Review.* 2015;65(2):275, 283.
5. Woolf SH. Progress in achieving health equity requires attention to root causes. *Health Affairs.* June 2017;36(6):984–991.
6. Weil AR. Pursuing health equity. *Health Affairs.* June 2017;36(6):975.

Index

Page numbers followed by *b, f,* or *t* indicate material in boxes, figures, or tables, respectively.